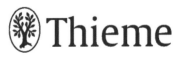

Decision Making in Orthopaedic Trauma

Meir T. Marmor, MD
Orthopaedic Trauma Institute
UCSF Department of Orthopaedic Surgery
Zuckerberg San Francisco General Hospital and Trauma Center
San Francisco, California

39 illustrations

Thieme
New York · Stuttgart · Delhi · Rio de Janeiro

Executive Editor: William Lamsback
Managing Editor: Nikole Y. Connors
Director, Editorial Services: Mary Jo Casey
Production Editor: Torsten Scheihagen
International Production Director: Andreas Schabert
International Marketing Director: Fiona Henderson
International Sales Director: Louisa Turrell
Director of Sales, North America: Mike Roseman
Senior Vice President and Chief Operating
Officer: Sarah Vanderbilt
President: Brian D. Scanlan
Printer: Everbest Printing Co.
Medical Illustrator: Andrea Hines
Algorithm Drawings: Andy Ma

Library of Congress Cataloging-in-Publication Data
Names: Marmor, Meir, editor.
Title: Decision making in orthopaedic trauma /
    [edited by] Meir Marmor, MD,
    Orthopaedic Trauma Institute,
    University of California San Francisco
    Department of Orthopaedic Surgery, Zuckerberg San Francisco
    General Hospital and Trauma Center, San Francisco, California.
Description: First edition. | New York : Thieme, 2017. |
        Includes bibliographical references.
Identifiers: LCCN 2017005102 (print) | LCCN 2017006617 (ebook) |
        ISBN 9781626234611 (print) |
        ISBN 9781626234628 (e-book)
Subjects: LCSH: Orthopaedics—Handbooks, manuals, etc. |
        Wounds and injuries—Surgery—Handbooks, manuals, etc.
Classification: LCC RD732.5 .D43 2017 (print) |
        LCC RD732.5 (ebook) | DDC 616.7—dc23
LC record available at https://lccn.loc.gov/2017005102

Thieme Publishers New York
333 Seventh Avenue, New York, NY 10001 USA
+1 800 782 3488, customerservice@thieme.com

Thieme Publishers Stuttgart
Rüdigerstrasse 14, 70469 Stuttgart, Germany
+49 [0]711 8931 421, customerservice@thieme.de

Thieme Publishers Delhi
A-12, Second Floor, Sector-2, Noida-201301
Uttar Pradesh, India
+91 120 45 566 00, customerservice@thieme.in

Thieme Publishers Rio de Janeiro, Thieme Publicações Ltda.
Edifício Rodolpho de Paoli, 25⁰ andar
Av. Nilo Peçanha, 50 – Sala 2508
Rio de Janeiro 20020-906 Brasil
+55 21 3172-2297 / +55 21 3172-1896

Cover design: Thieme Publishing Group
Typesetting by DiTech Process Solutions

Printed in China by Everbest Printing Co.   5 4 3 2 1

ISBN 978-1-62623-461-1

Also available as an e-book:
eISBN 978-1-62623-462-8

Important note: Medicine is an ever-changing science undergoing continual development. Research and clinical experience are continually expanding our knowledge, in particular our knowledge of proper treatment and drug therapy. Insofar as this book mentions any dosage or application, readers may rest assured that the authors, editors, and publishers have made every effort to ensure that such references are in accordance with **the state of knowledge at the time of production of the book.**

Nevertheless, this does not involve, imply, or express any guarantee or responsibility on the part of the publishers in respect to any dosage instructions and forms of applications stated in the book. **Every user is requested to examine carefully** the manufacturers' leaflets accompanying each drug and to check, if necessary in consultation with a physician or specialist, whether the dosage schedules mentioned therein or the contraindications stated by the manufacturers differ from the statements made in the present book. Such examination is particularly important with drugs that are either rarely used or have been newly released on the market. Every dosage schedule or every form of application used is entirely at the user's own risk and responsibility. The authors and publishers request every user to report to the publishers any discrepancies or inaccuracies noticed. If errors in this work are found after publication, errata will be posted at www.thieme.com on the product description page.

Some of the product names, patents, and registered designs referred to in this book are in fact registered trademarks or proprietary names even though specific reference to this fact is not always made in the text. Therefore, the appearance of a name without designation as proprietary is not to be construed as a representation by the publisher that it is in the public domain.

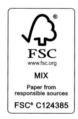

To my wife and children who put up with me with endless patience, and to the future orthopaedic trauma patients who will benefit from this book.

Contents

Contents

Contents

Preface

"Truth is ever to be found in simplicity, and not in the multiplicity and confusion of things."

—Isaac Newton

"Simplicity is the ultimate sophistication."

—Leonardo da Vinci

Expecting the unexpected is the hallmark of trauma management. When dealing with orthopaedic trauma, one not only needs to deal with the unexpected, but also to have an understanding of a great number of complex of injuries and an ever-growing number of available treatments. Surgeons, physicians, nurses, therapists, and medical staff who treat musculoskeletal injuries need to have a common language and understanding of the critical decisions and management options for the various injuries. However, this information is not easy to come by. The information age in medicine has flooded the medical community with data on the effectiveness of medical treatments. At the same time, the demand for evidence-based medicine has increased the quality and sophistication of medical research, making the interpretation of medical research a task for the experts. Existing websites and textbooks are not always approachable to the non-expert orthopaedic trauma surgeon and often lack the simplicity to become useful for a large audience. In some instances, a caregiver treating orthopaedic injuries only wants to ask an expert in the field, "What would you do for these kinds of injuries?" That is where this book comes in. Rather that offering an exhaustive list of all the options of treating a given injury, the reader can quickly understand the most critical decisions and treatment options for the most common orthopaedic injuries. All of the chapters in this book were written by experts in the field of orthopaedic trauma and perioperative care, all of them working in the Orthopaedic Trauma Institute.

The Orthopaedic Trauma Institute (OTI) is a collaboration between the University of California, San Francisco (UCSF) and the Zuckerberg San Francisco General (ZSFG) Hospital and Trauma Center. The OTI is the only trauma center in San Francisco specializing in the treatment and rehabilitation of musculoskeletal injuries. The Institute provides expert care for all aspects of traumatic musculoskeletal injuries, including inpatient and outpatient orthopaedic surgical care, rehabilitation, and orthotics and prosthetics. Surgeons and physicians from the Department of Orthopaedic Surgery at UCSF with specific training and experience in treating these conditions staff the OTI. Since 2005, the OTI has put on the largest annual orthopaedic trauma surgical course in the United States, drawing instructors and attendees from over 20 countries and 40 states each year. The OTI staff also founded the Institute for Global Orthopaedics and Traumatology, which carries the global educational work of the OTI. The clinical, educational, global work and research done in the OTI, all lend themselves to the fulfillment of the OTI mission: "To mend the injured, inspire innovators, and empower leaders to restore lives."

The chapters in this book are not a substitute for detailed, comprehensive protocols of management of the various musculoskeletal conditions listed in this book. The chapters try to distil the critical decisions needed to manage each injury. Although they are not replacements for protocols, they can form the basis for such protocols, and any protocol on a given subject will likely need to address the critical decision making showcased in this book. The book chapters are not a final word, but a snapshot of an acceptable current approach to management of a specific injury according to the understanding of contemporary biomedical research and personal experience of the chapter's author. Although largely literature based, the chapters are subjective by nature, and can only answer one question: "What would this given expert do for these types of injuries?" An effort was made to include in each chapter the pertinent imaging (dark gray blocks), decisions to be made (maroon hexagons), actions to be taken (light blue blocks) and non-operative/rehabilitation treatments (purple blocks). To aid in the understanding of the decision trees, information blocks, tables, figures, images, and abbreviation indexes were added as needed. Additionally, the authors were instructed to attach suggested readings to whenever these readings directly contribute to their decision-making process. For the most part, the chapters are arranged according to anatomic location, with general orthopaedic trauma subjects and perioperative care chapters in the beginning of the book and pathologic fractures and fracture complications at the end. To ease the finding of information, appendices summarizing the imaging, non-operative treatments, rehabilitation, and common orthotics in use for the various injuries were added. An additional appendix on a potential method for estimating time to return to work for an orthopaedic trauma patient was added as well. The readers are encouraged to add their comments to the decision trees and to tailor them to their specific workplace and patient population. We at the OTI welcome any comments on the decision-making processes or suggestions about studies that can change any of the decisions outlined in this book. These comments or suggestions can be sent directly to me (meir.marmor@ucsf.edu).

Meir T. Marmor, MD

Acknowledgments

I would like to thank my fellow co-workers at the Orthopaedic Trauma Institute (OTI), at the Zuckerberg San Francisco Hospital and Trauma Center, at Regional Medical Center of San Jose, and at Enloe Medical Center in Chico for making my daily work so enjoyable and inspiring me to make this book.

Contributors

Richard Coughlin, MD, MSc
Orthopaedic Trauma Institute
UCSF Department of Orthopaedic Surgery
Zuckerberg San Francisco General Hospital and
Trauma Center
San Francisco, California

Aarti Deshpande, CPO
Orthopaedic Trauma Institute
UCSF Department of Orthopaedic Surgery
Zuckerberg San Francisco General Hospital and
Trauma Center
San Francisco, California

Harry Jergesen, MD
Orthopaedic Trauma Institute
UCSF Department of Orthopaedic Surgery
Zuckerberg San Francisco General Hospital and
Trauma Center
San Francisco, California

Utku Kandemir, MD
Orthopaedic Trauma Institute
UCSF Department of Orthopaedic Surgery
Zuckerberg San Francisco General Hospital and
Trauma Center
San Francisco, California

Jeremie Larouche, MD
Orthopaedic Trauma Institute
UCSF Department of Orthopaedic Surgery
Zuckerberg San Francisco General Hospital and
Trauma Center
San Francisco, California

Nicolas Lee, MD
Orthopaedic Trauma Institute
UCSF Department of Orthopaedic Surgery
Zuckerberg San Francisco General Hospital and
Trauma Center
San Francisco, California

Meir T. Marmor, MD
Orthopaedic Trauma Institute
UCSF Department of Orthopaedic Surgery
Zuckerberg San Francisco General Hospital and
Trauma Center
San Francisco, California

Amir Matityahu, MD
Orthopaedic Trauma Institute
UCSF Department of Orthopaedic Surgery
Zuckerberg San Francisco General Hospital and
Trauma Center
San Francisco, California

R. Trigg McClellan, MD
Orthopaedic Trauma Institute
UCSF Department of Orthopaedic Surgery
Zuckerberg San Francisco General Hospital and
Trauma Center
San Francisco, California

Eric Meinberg, MD
Orthopaedic Trauma Institute
UCSF Department of Orthopaedic Surgery
Zuckerberg San Francisco General Hospital and
Trauma Center
San Francisco, California

Ben Mellott, PT
Physical Therapy Department
Zuckerberg San Francisco General Hospital and
Trauma Center
San Francisco, California

Theodore Miclau, MD
Orthopaedic Trauma Institute
UCSF Department of Orthopaedic Surgery
Zuckerberg San Francisco General Hospital and
Trauma Center
San Francisco, California

Saam Morshed, MD, PhD
Orthopaedic Trauma Institute
UCSF Department of Orthopaedic Surgery
Zuckerberg San Francisco General Hospital and
Trauma Center
San Francisco, California

Masato Nagao, MD, PhD
Orthopaedic Trauma Institute
UCSF Department of Orthopaedic Surgery
Zuckerberg San Francisco General Hospital and
Trauma Center
San Francisco, California

Lisa Pascual, MD
Orthopaedic Trauma Institute
UCSF Department of Orthopaedic Surgery
Zuckerberg San Francisco General Hospital and
Trauma Center
San Francisco, California

Nicole Schroeder, MD
Orthopaedic Trauma Institute
UCSF Department of Orthopaedic Surgery
Zuckerberg San Francisco General Hospital and
Trauma Center
San Francisco, California

Dave Shearer, MD
Orthopaedic Trauma Institute
UCSF Department of Orthopaedic Surgery
Zuckerberg San Francisco General Hospital and
Trauma Center
San Francisco, California

Paul Toogood, MD
Orthopaedic Trauma Institute
UCSF Department of Orthopaedic Surgery
Zuckerberg San Francisco General Hospital and
Trauma Center
San Francisco, California

Rosanna Wustrack, MD
Orthopaedic Trauma Institute
UCSF Department of Orthopaedic Surgery
Zuckerberg San Francisco General Hospital and
Trauma Center
San Francisco, California

Decision Making in
Orthopaedic Trauma

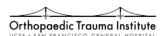

Orthopaedic Trauma Institute
UCSF + SAN FRANCISCO GENERAL HOSPITAL

Meir T. Marmor, MD

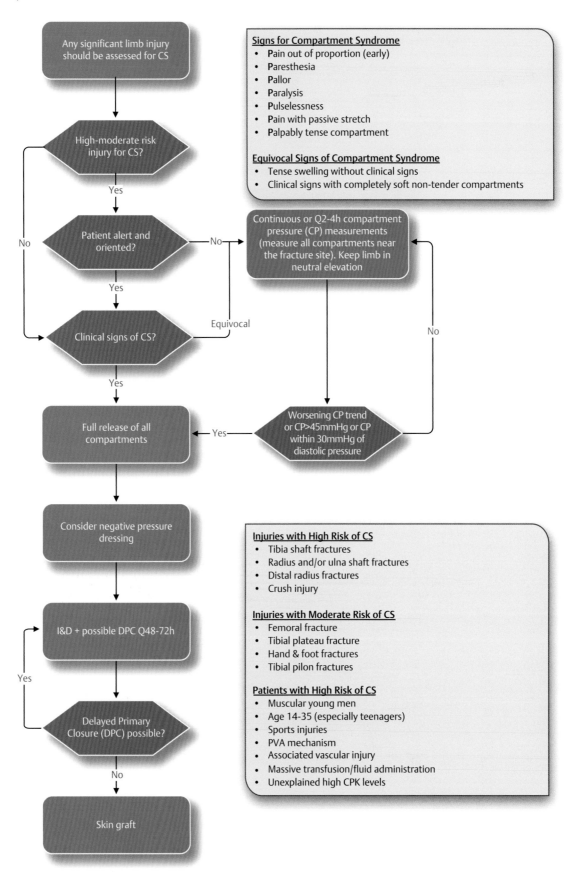

Any significant limb injury should be assessed for CS

Signs for Compartment Syndrome
- Pain out of proportion (early)
- Paresthesia
- Pallor
- Paralysis
- Pulselessness
- Pain with passive stretch
- Palpably tense compartment

Equivocal Signs of Compartment Syndrome
- Tense swelling without clinical signs
- Clinical signs with completely soft non-tender compartments

High-moderate risk injury for CS? — No

Yes

Patient alert and oriented? — No → Continuous or Q2-4h compartment pressure (CP) measurements (measure all compartments near the fracture site). Keep limb in neutral elevation

Yes

Clinical signs of CS? — Equivocal

Yes

No

Full release of all compartments ← Yes — Worsening CP trend or CP>45mmHg or CP within 30mmHg of diastolic pressure — No

Consider negative pressure dressing

Injuries with High Risk of CS
- Tibia shaft fractures
- Radius and/or ulna shaft fractures
- Distal radius fractures
- Crush injury

Injuries with Moderate Risk of CS
- Femoral fracture
- Tibial plateau fracture
- Hand & foot fractures
- Tibial pilon fractures

Patients with High Risk of CS
- Muscular young men
- Age 14-35 (especially teenagers)
- Sports injuries
- PVA mechanism
- Associated vascular injury
- Massive transfusion/fluid administration
- Unexplained high CPK levels

I&D + possible DPC Q48-72h

Yes

Delayed Primary Closure (DPC) possible?

No

Skin graft

Suggested Readings

McQueen MM, Gaston P, Court-Brown CM. Acute compartment syndrome. Who is at risk? J Bone Joint Surg Br 2000;82(2):200–203

McQueen MM, Duckworth AD. The diagnosis of acute compartment syndrome: a review. Eur J Trauma Emerg Surg 2014;40(5):521–528

McQueen MM, Duckworth AD, Aitken SA, Court-Brown CM. The estimated sensitivity and specificity of compartment pressure monitoring for acute compartment syndrome. J Bone Joint Surg Am 2013;95(8):673–677

McQueen MM, Court-Brown CM. Compartment monitoring in tibial fractures. The pressure threshold for decompression. J Bone Joint Surg Br 1996;78(1):99–104

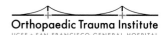
Meir T. Marmor, MD

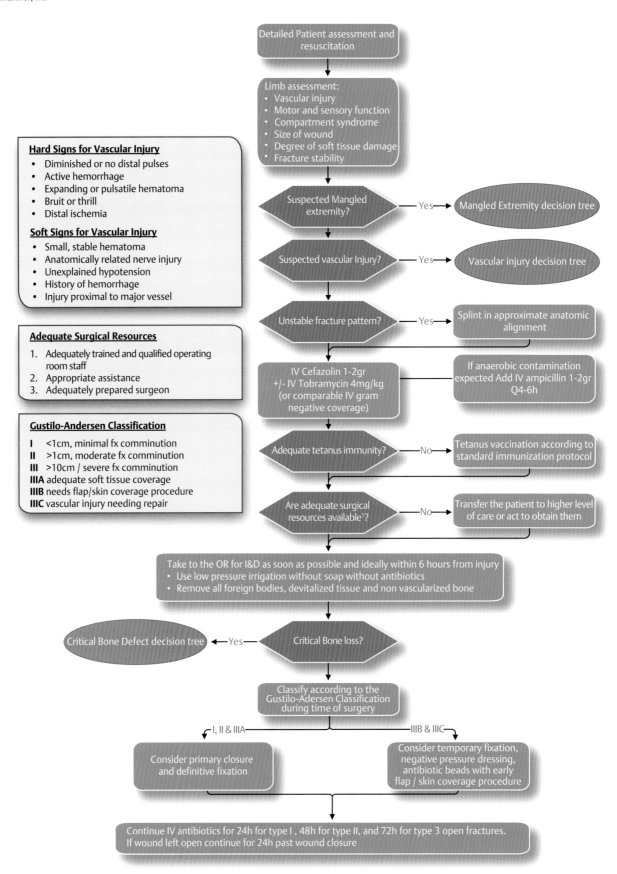

Hard Signs for Vascular Injury
- Diminished or no distal pulses
- Active hemorrhage
- Expanding or pulsatile hematoma
- Bruit or thrill
- Distal ischemia

Soft Signs for Vascular Injury
- Small, stable hematoma
- Anatomically related nerve injury
- Unexplained hypotension
- History of hemorrhage
- Injury proximal to major vessel

Adequate Surgical Resources
1. Adequately trained and qualified operating room staff
2. Appropriate assistance
3. Adequately prepared surgeon

Gustilo-Andersen Classification

I   <1cm, minimal fx comminution
II >1cm, moderate fx comminution
III >10cm / severe fx comminution
IIIA adequate soft tissue coverage
IIIB needs flap/skin coverage procedure
IIIC vascular injury needing repair

Detailed Patient assessment and resuscitation

Limb assessment:
- Vascular injury
- Motor and sensory function
- Compartment syndrome
- Size of wound
- Degree of soft tissue damage
- Fracture stability

Suspected Mangled extremity? —Yes→ Mangled Extremity decision tree

Suspected vascular Injury? —Yes→ Vascular injury decision tree

Unstable fracture pattern? —Yes→ Splint in approximate anatomic alignment

IV Cefazolin 1-2gr +/- IV Tobramycin 4mg/kg (or comparable IV gram negative coverage) — If anaerobic contamination expected Add IV ampicillin 1-2gr Q4-6h

Adequate tetanus immunity? —No→ Tetanus vaccination according to standard immunization protocol

Are adequate surgical resources available[1]? —No→ Transfer the patient to higher level of care or act to obtain them

Take to the OR for I&D as soon as possible and ideally within 6 hours from injury
- Use low pressure irrigation without soap without antibiotics
- Remove all foreign bodies, devitalized tissue and non vascularized bone

Critical Bone Defect decision tree ←Yes— Critical Bone loss?

Classify according to the Gustilo-Adersen Classification during time of surgery

I, II & IIIA — Consider primary closure and definitive fixation

IIIB & IIIC — Consider temporary fixation, negative pressure dressing, antibiotic beads with early flap / skin coverage procedure

Continue IV antibiotics for 24h for type I , 48h for type II, and 72h for type 3 open fractures. If wound left open continue for 24h past wound closure

Suggested Readings

Pollak AN, Jones AL, Castillo RC, Bosse MJ, MacKenzie EJ; LEAP Study Group. The relationship between time to surgical debridement and incidence of infection after open high-energy lower extremity trauma. J Bone Joint Surg Am 2010;92(1):7–15

Zalavras CG, Marcus RE, Levin LS, Patzakis MJ. Management of open fractures and subsequent complications. J Bone Joint Surg Am 2007;89(4):884–895

Bhandari M, Jeray KJ, Petrisor BA, et al; FLOW Investigators. A Trial of Wound Irrigation in the Initial Management of Open Fracture Wounds. N Engl J Med 2015;373(27):2629–2641

Gustilo RB, Anderson JT. Prevention of infection in the treatment of one thousand and twenty-five open fractures of long bones: retrospective and prospective analyses. J Bone Joint Surg Am 1976;58(4):453–458

Fischer MD, Gustilo RB, Varecka TF. The timing of flap coverage, bone-grafting, and intramedullary nailing in patients who have a fracture of the tibial shaft with extensive soft-tissue injury. J Bone Joint Surg Am 1991;73(9):1316–1322

Chapter 3: Ballistic Injuries

Paul Toogood, MD

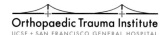

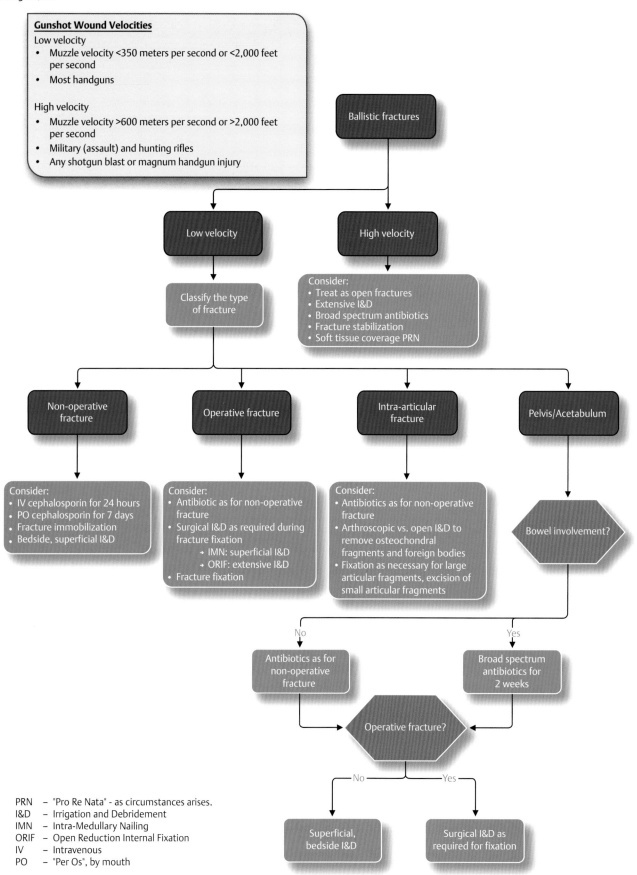

Gunshot Wound Velocities

Low velocity
- Muzzle velocity <350 meters per second or <2,000 feet per second
- Most handguns

High velocity
- Muzzle velocity >600 meters per second or >2,000 feet per second
- Military (assault) and hunting rifles
- Any shotgun blast or magnum handgun injury

Ballistic fractures

Low velocity

High velocity

Classify the type of fracture

Consider:
- Treat as open fractures
- Extensive I&D
- Broad spectrum antibiotics
- Fracture stabilization
- Soft tissue coverage PRN

Non-operative fracture

Operative fracture

Intra-articular fracture

Pelvis/Acetabulum

Consider:
- IV cephalosporin for 24 hours
- PO cephalosporin for 7 days
- Fracture immobilization
- Bedside, superficial I&D

Consider:
- Antibiotic as for non-operative fracture
- Surgical I&D as required during fracture fixation
  → IMN: superficial I&D
  → ORIF: extensive I&D
- Fracture fixation

Consider:
- Antibiotics as for non-operative fracture
- Arthroscopic vs. open I&D to remove osteochondral fragments and foreign bodies
- Fixation as necessary for large articular fragments, excision of small articular fragments

Bowel involvement?

No

Yes

Antibiotics as for non-operative fracture

Broad spectrum antibiotics for 2 weeks

Operative fracture?

No

Yes

Superficial, bedside I&D

Surgical I&D as required for fixation

PRN – "Pro Re Nata" - as circumstances arises.
I&D – Irrigation and Debridement
IMN – Intra-Medullary Nailing
ORIF – Open Reduction Internal Fixation
IV – Intravenous
PO – "Per Os", by mouth

Suggested Readings

Sathiyakumar V, Thakore RV, Stinner DJ, Obremskey WT, Ficke JR, Sethi MK. Gunshot-induced fractures of the extremities: a review of antibiotic and debridement practices. Curr Rev Musculoskelet Med 2015;8(3):276–289

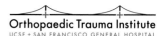

Orthopaedic Trauma Institute
UCSF + SAN FRANCISCO GENERAL HOSPITAL

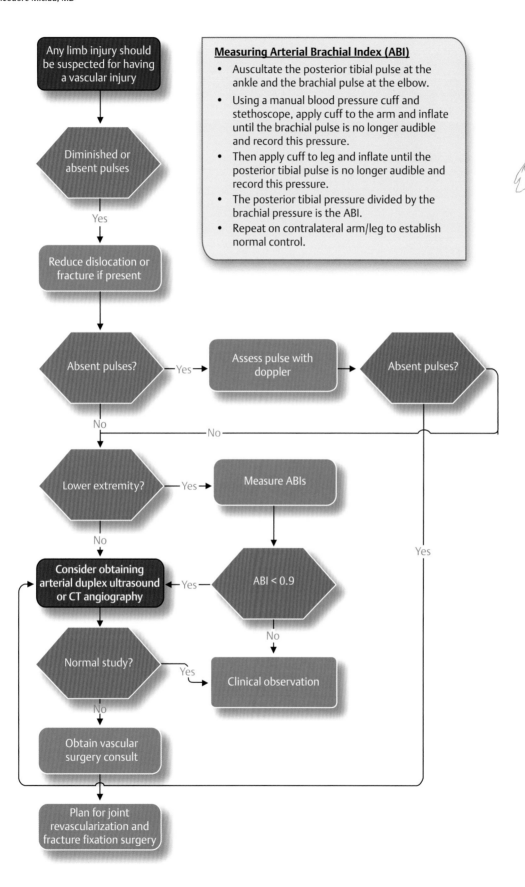

Any limb injury should be suspected for having a vascular injury

Diminished or absent pulses

Yes

Reduce dislocation or fracture if present

Measuring Arterial Brachial Index (ABI)
- Auscultate the posterior tibial pulse at the ankle and the brachial pulse at the elbow.
- Using a manual blood pressure cuff and stethoscope, apply cuff to the arm and inflate until the brachial pulse is no longer audible and record this pressure.
- Then apply cuff to leg and inflate until the posterior tibial pulse is no longer audible and record this pressure.
- The posterior tibial pressure divided by the brachial pressure is the ABI.
- Repeat on contralateral arm/leg to establish normal control.

Absent pulses? — Yes → Assess pulse with doppler → Absent pulses?

No

No

Lower extremity? — Yes → Measure ABIs

No

Consider obtaining arterial duplex ultrasound or CT angiography ← Yes — ABI < 0.9

Yes

No

Normal study? — Yes → Clinical observation

No

Obtain vascular surgery consult

Plan for joint revascularization and fracture fixation surgery

Suggested Readings

Mills WJ, Barei DP, McNair P. The value of the ankle–brachial index for diagnosing arterial injury after knee dislocation: a prospective study. Journal of Trauma and Acute Care Surgery. 2004 Jun 1;56(6):1261-5.

Chapter 5: Traumatic Nerve Injury

Masato Nagao, MD, PhD

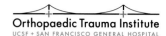
Orthopaedic Trauma Institute
UCSF + SAN FRANCISCO GENERAL HOSPITAL

Seddon	Sunderland	Pathology
Neurapraxia	1st Degree	Conduction block and demyelination
Axonotmesis	2nd Degree	Axon Loss Endoneurium, perineurium and epineurium intact
	3rd Degree	Axon Loss Endoneurium disrupted Perineurium and epineurium intact
	4th Degree	Axon Loss Endoneurium and perineurium disrupted Epineurium intact
Neurotmesis	5th Degree	Axon Loss Endoneurium, perineurium and epineurium disrupted

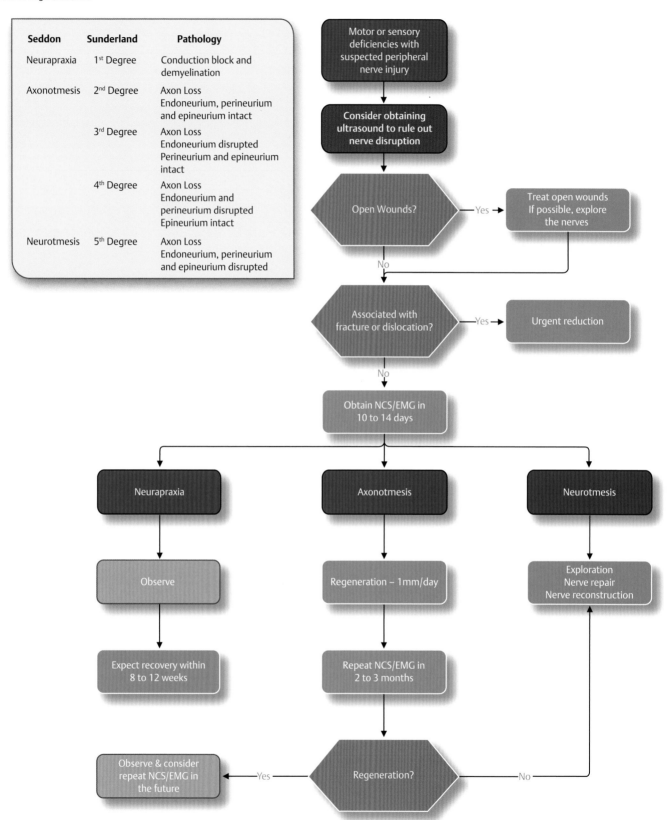

NCS – Nerve Conduction Study
EMG – Electromyography

Suggested Readings

Seddon HJ. Three types of nerve injury. Brain 1943;66(4):237–288

Sunderland S. A classification of peripheral nerve injuries producing loss of function. Brain 1951;74(4):491–516

Sunderland S. The anatomy and physiology of nerve injury. Muscle Nerve 1990;13(9):771–784

Robinson LR. How electrodiagnosis predicts clinical outcome of focal peripheral nerve lesions. Muscle Nerve 2015; 52 (3): 321-333

Robinson LR. Traumatic injury to peripheral nerves. Muscle Nerve 2000;23(6):863–873

Campbell WW. Evaluation and management of peripheral nerve injury. Clin Neurophysiol 2008;119(9):1951–1965

Theodore Miclau, MD

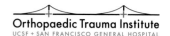

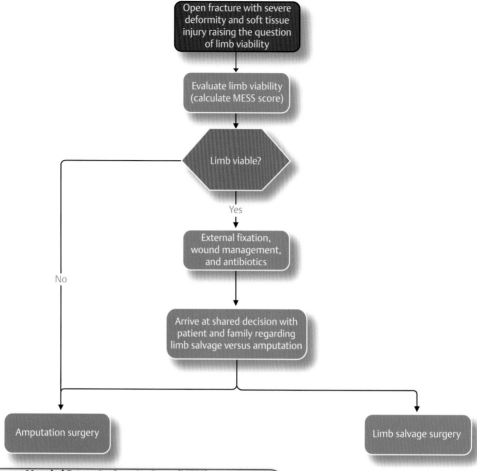

Mangled Extremity Severity Score (MESS)			
Type	**Characteristics**	**Injury**	**Points**
1	Low energy	Stab wound, simple closed fractures, small-caliber GSW	1
2	Medium energy	Open/multilevel fractures, dislocation, moderate crush	2
3	High energy	Shotgun, high-velocity GSW	3
4	Massive crush	Logging, railroad, oil rig accidents	4
Shock Group			
1	Normotensive	BP stable	0
2	Transiently hypotensive	BP unstable in field but responsive to fluid	1
3	Prolonged hypotension	SBP <80 mmHg in field and responsive to IV fluids in OR	2
Ischemia Group			
1	None	Pulsatile, no signs of ischemia	1
2	Mild	Diminished pulses without signs of ischemia	2
3	Moderate	No dopplerable pulse, sluggish cap refill, paresthesia, diminished motor activity	3
4	Advanced	Pulseless, cool, paralyzed, numb without cap refill	4
Age Group			
1	<30 year old		0
2	>30 <50		1
Calculate MESS by adding the score from each category. MESS <=6 is consistent with a salvageable limb			

Key Results of LEAP Study

- Sickness Impact Profile and return to work is not significantly different between amputation and reconstruction at 2 years.
- Loss of plantar sensation is not a contraindication for reconstruction

Suggested Readings

Bosse MJ, MacKenzie EJ, Kellam JF, et al. An analysis of outcomes of reconstruction or amputation after leg-threatening injuries. N Engl J Med 2002;347(24):1924–1931

Busse JW, Jacobs CL, Swiontkowski MF, Bosse MJ, Bhandari M; Evidence-Based Orthopaedic Trauma Working Group. Complex limb salvage or early amputation for severe lower-limb injury: a meta-analysis of observational studies. J Orthop Trauma 2007;21(1):70–76

Helfet DL, Howey T, Sanders R, Johansen K. Limb salvage versus amputation. Preliminary results of the Mangled Extremity Severity Score. Clin Orthop Relat Res 1990; (256):80–86

Chapter 7: Polytrauma Patient

Saam Morshed, MD, PhD

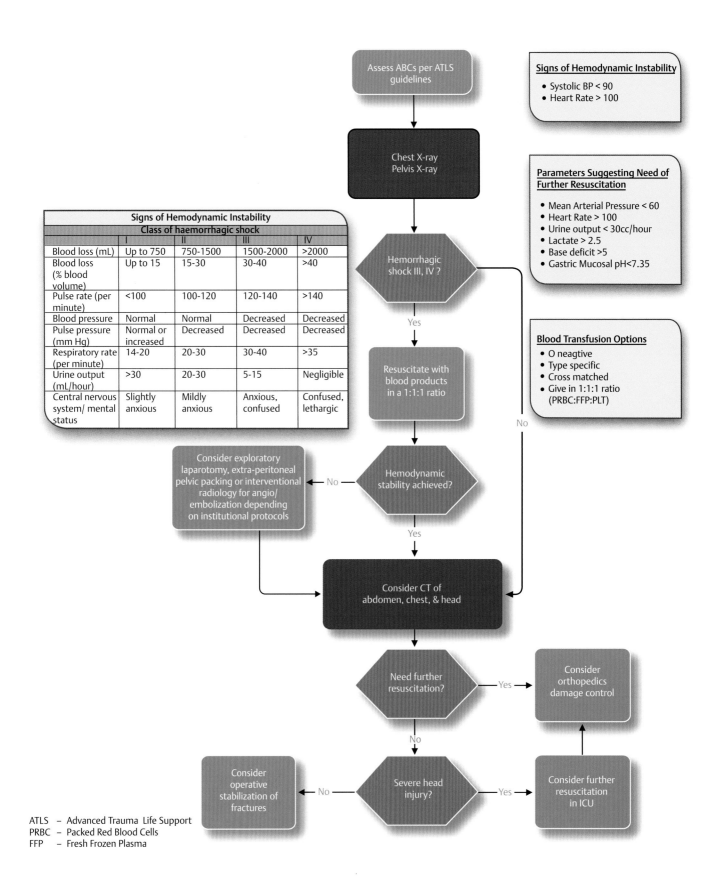

Signs of Hemodynamic Instability
- Systolic BP < 90
- Heart Rate > 100

Parameters Suggesting Need of Further Resuscitation
- Mean Arterial Pressure < 60
- Heart Rate > 100
- Urine output < 30cc/hour
- Lactate > 2.5
- Base deficit >5
- Gastric Mucosal pH<7.35

Blood Transfusion Options
- O neagtive
- Type specific
- Cross matched
- Give in 1:1:1 ratio (PRBC:FFP:PLT)

Assess ABCs per ATLS guidelines

Chest X-ray Pelvis X-ray

Hemorrhagic shock III, IV ?

Resuscitate with blood products in a 1:1:1 ratio

Consider exploratory laparotomy, extra-peritoneal pelvic packing or interventional radiology for angio/ embolization depending on institutional protocols

Hemodynamic stability achieved?

Consider CT of abdomen, chest, & head

Need further resuscitation?

Consider orthopedics damage control

Consider operative stabilization of fractures

Severe head injury?

Consider further resuscitation in ICU

Signs of Hemodynamic Instability				
Class of haemorrhagic shock				
	I	II	III	IV
Blood loss (mL)	Up to 750	750-1500	1500-2000	>2000
Blood loss (% blood volume)	Up to 15	15-30	30-40	>40
Pulse rate (per minute)	<100	100-120	120-140	>140
Blood pressure	Normal	Normal	Decreased	Decreased
Pulse pressure (mm Hg)	Normal or increased	Decreased	Decreased	Decreased
Respiratory rate (per minute)	14-20	20-30	30-40	>35
Urine output (mL/hour)	>30	20-30	5-15	Negligible
Central nervous system/ mental status	Slightly anxious	Mildly anxious	Anxious, confused	Confused, lethargic

ATLS – Advanced Trauma Life Support
PRBC – Packed Red Blood Cells
FFP – Fresh Frozen Plasma

Suggested Readings

Pape HC, Giannoudis P, Krettek C. The timing of fracture treatment in polytrauma patients: relevance of damage control orthopedic surgery. Am J Surg 2002;183(6):622–629

ATLS Subcommittee; American College of Surgeons' Committee on Trauma; International ATLS working group. Advanced trauma life support (ATLS®): the ninth edition. J Trauma Acute Care Surg 2013;74(5):1363–1366

Holcomb JB, Tilley BC, Baraniuk S, et al; PROPPR Study Group. Transfusion of plasma, platelets, and red blood cells in a 1:1:1 vs a 1:1:2 ratio and mortality in patients with severe trauma: the PROPPR randomized clinical trial. JAMA 2015;313(5):471–482

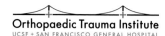
Lisa Pascual, MD

Oral Long Acting Opioid of Choice

- Do not exceed 3 gm of acetaminophen (APAP) / 24 hours
- APAP (300 mg) + codeine 15 mg (#2), 30 mg (#3), 60 mg (#4) q4h
- Vicodin (5 mg hydrocodone + 500 mg APAP) q4h
- Norco or Lortab (5 mg or 7.5 mg or 10 mg + 325 mg APAP) q4-6h
- Percocet (2.5 mg or 5 mg or 7.5 mg or 10 mg oxycodone + 325 APAP) q6h

Stool Softener of Choice

- Diet (postop): fiber, water, prune juice
- Supp/Tab – Bisacodyl (Dulcolax) 10mg (5-15mg) q24h
- Cap/Sol/Syr Docusate (Colace) 200mg (50-500mg) q24h or divided q6h/q12
- Tab/Sol Senna (Senokot) 15-25mg qHS (up to 2/d)
- Milk of magnesia 30-60mL/d (reg) 10 30mL/d(concentrated)

Acetaminophen (APAP) Dosages:

Weight >=50 kg:
Parenteral (IV):
- IV 1000mg Q6h OR IV 650 mg Q4h
- PO 325-1000mg Q4-6h

Maximum Single Dose: 1000 mg
Minimum Dosing Interval: every 4 hours
Maximum Dose: 4000 mg/ 24 hours
(3000mg/24 hours is ideal)

Weight < 50 kg:
- IV/PO 15 mg/kg Q6h OR 12.5 mg/kg IV Q4h

Maximum Single Dose: 15 mg/kg
Minimum Dosing Interval: every 4 hours
Maximum Dose: 75 mg/kg per 24 hours

APAP – Acetaminophen
NSAID – Nonsteroidal Anti-Inflammatory Drug

Flowchart

Patient with fracture is admitted to the hospital Fracture is splinted in the ER, limb is elevated and iced, consider regional block for hip fractures

→ Treat with short acting IV APAP and/or short acting IV opioid of choice

→ Treat with stool softener

→ Treat with IV anti-emetic

→ Is the patient at risk for stress ulcers?
- Yes → Start stress ulcer prevention with PPI (Omeprazole 20 mg daily) and H2 blocker (Famotidine 20 mg BID)
- No → Does patient need surgery?
  - Yes → Would patient benefit from a regional block? (if not already done)
    - Yes → Treat according to Regional Block algorithm
    - No → Surgery
    → Add PCA treatment if needed
  - No → Treat pain according to general principles utilizing "multimodal" analgesia

Surgery → (No) → Contraindications for PCA?

Contraindications for PCA?
- Yes → NSAIDS, antineuropathic and APAP treatment

After 24-48 hours calculate total use of opioids

→ Convert to long acting opioid and short acting opioid

→ Discontinue PCA if utilized

→ Plan for a narcotic tapering protocol over the first 2 weeks after surgery

Opioid Conversion Chart (equivalent doses)

Drug	Route	Dose
Morphine	IV	10mg
Morphine	PO	30mg
Dilaudid	IV	1.5mg
Dilaudid	PO	7.5mg
Oxycodone	PO	20mg
Percocet	PO	20mg
Hydrocodone	PO	30mg
Codeine	PO	200mg

General Principles

- If a patient reports he/she is in pain, then he/she is in pain
- Pain cannot be treated appropriately if it is not assessed and monitored for effects and side effects
- Analgesics are best given on a regular and not PRN basis
- For severe pain, consider IV analgesia

Short Acting IV Opiod of Choice (initial dose)

- Morphine, initial dose: 2.5mg IV
- Hydromorphone: 0.2-1mg IV
- Fentanyl 25mcg IV
- Consider dosage reduction in elderly

IV Anti-emetic of Choice

- Ondansetron (Zofran) 4mg Q8h PRN
- Promethazine (Phenergan) 6.25mg Q6h PRN
- Metocolopramide (Reglan) 10mg Q6h PRN

Patient Controlled Analgesia (PCA) of Choice

- Morphine PCA protocol
- Hydromorphone (Dilaudid) PCA

PCA Contraindications

- Inability to understand/use PCA
- Increased intra-cranial pressure
- Sleep apnea or respiratory compromise

NSAIDS of Choice

- IV Ketorolac (Toradol) 15mg Q6h
- Naproxen (Naprosyn) 500mg Q12h
- Ibuprofen (Motrin) 600mg Q6h
- + PPI: Omeprazole 20 mg daily

NSAIDS Contraindications (BARS)

- Bleeding (Coagulopathy)
- Asthma (10% of asthmatics)
- Renal Disease
- Stomach (peptic ulcer/gastritis)

Oral Long Acting Opioid of Choice

- Morphine (MS Contin) 15, 30, 60, 100 Q12h
- Oxycodone (Oxycontin) CR 10mg Q8-12h (10,20,40,80mg)

Antineuropathic of Choice

- Gabapentin
- Pregabalin

Suggested Readings

Boursinos LA, Karachalios T, Poultsides L, Malizos KN. Do steroids, conventional non-steroidal anti-inflammatory drugs and selective Cox-2 inhibitors adversely affect fracture healing? J Musculoskelet Neuronal Interact 2009;9(1):44–52

Chang AK, Bijur PE, Daviit M, Gallagher JE. Randomized clinical trial of an intravenous hydromorphone titration intravenous hydromorphone titration protocol versuis usual care for mangement of acute pain in older emergency department patients. Drugs Aging 2013;30(9):747–754

Chang AK, Bijur PE, Gallagher EJ. Randomized clinical trial comparing the safety and efficacy of a hydromorphone titration protocol to usual care in the management of adult emergency department patients with acute severe pain. Ann Emerg Med 2011;58(4):352–359

DeVellis P, Thomas SH, Wedel SK. Prehospital and emergency department analgesia for air-transported patients with fractures. Prehosp Emerg Care 1998;2(4):293–296

Gandhi K, Viscusi E. Multimodal pain management techniques in hip and knee arthroplasty. The Journal of New York School of Regional Anesthesia 2009;13:1–9

Hudcova J, Mcnicol ED, Quah CS, Carr DB. Patient controlled opioid anagesia versus conventional opioid analgesia for postoperative pain. (review) Cochrane Libr 2012

Jin F, Chung F. Multimodal analgesia for postoperative pain control. J Clin Anesth 2001;13(7):524–539

Kolber MR, Lindblad AJ, Taylor IC. We stand by our conclusion. Can Fam Physician 2015;61(1):25

Wright JM, Price SD, Watson WA. NSAID use and efficacy in the emergency department: single doses of oral ibuprofen versus intramuscular ketorolac. Ann Pharmacother 1994;28(3):309–312

Lucas SD, Le-Windling L, Enneking FK. Regional anesthesia for the trauma patient. Pain Management - Current Issues and Opinions. 2012. ISBN: 978-953-307-813-7. http://www.intechopen.com/books/pain-management-current-issues-and-opinions/regional-anesthesia-forthe-trauma-patient

Riddell M, Ospina M, Holroyd-Leduc JM. Use of femoral nerve blocks to manage hip fracture pain among older adults in the emergency department: A systematic review. Canadian Journal of Emergency Medicine, FirstView 2015; 1–8

Ritcey B, Pageau P, Woo MY, Perry JJ. Regional nerve blocks for hip and femoral neck fractures in the emergency department: A systematic review. Canadian Journal of Emergency Medicine, FirstView 2015; 1–11

Thomas SH. Fentanyl in the prehospital setting. Am J Emerg Med 2007;25(7):842–843

Turturro MA, Paris PM, Seaberg DC. Intramuscular ketorolac versus oral ibuprofen in acute musculoskeletal pain. Ann Emerg Med 1995;26(2):117–120

Vadivelu N, Mitra S, Narayan D. Recent advances in postoperative pain management. Yale J Biol Med 2010;83(1):11–25

Chapter 9: Chronic Pain Management

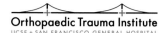
Orthopaedic Trauma Institute
UCSF + SAN FRANCISCO GENERAL HOSPITAL

Lisa Pascual, MD

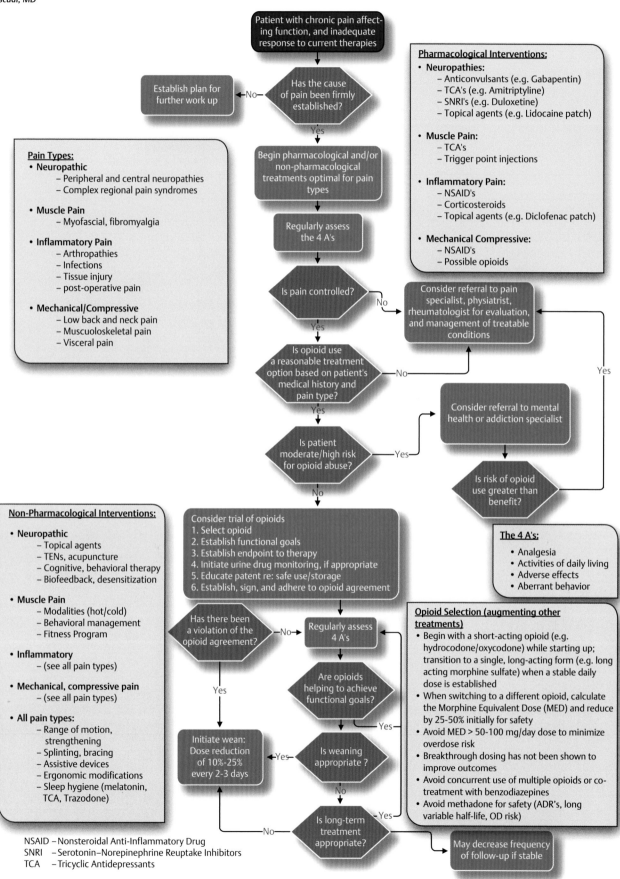

Patient with chronic pain affecting function, and inadequate response to current therapies

Has the cause of pain been firmly established?
— No → **Establish plan for further work up**

Yes ↓

Begin pharmacological and/or non-pharmacological treatments optimal for pain types

Regularly assess the 4 A's

Is pain controlled?
— No → **Consider referral to pain specialist, physiatrist, rheumatologist for evaluation, and management of treatable conditions**

Yes ↓

Is opioid use a reasonable treatment option based on patient's medical history and pain type?
— No →

Yes ↓

Is patient moderate/high risk for opioid abuse?
— Yes → **Consider referral to mental health or addiction specialist**

Is risk of opioid use greater than benefit?
— Yes →

No ↓

Consider trial of opioids
1. Select opioid
2. Establish functional goals
3. Establish endpoint to therapy
4. Initiate urine drug monitoring, if appropriate
5. Educate patent re: safe use/storage
6. Establish, sign, and adhere to opioid agreement

Has there been a violation of the opioid agreement?
— No → **Regularly assess 4 A's**
— Yes ↓

Are opioids helping to achieve functional goals?
— Yes →

Initiate wean: Dose reduction of 10%-25% every 2-3 days
← Yes — **Is weaning appropriate ?**

No ↓

Is long-term treatment appropriate?
— Yes →
— No →

May decrease frequency of follow-up if stable

Pain Types:
- **Neuropathic**
  - Peripheral and central neuropathies
  - Complex regional pain syndromes
- **Muscle Pain**
  - Myofascial, fibromyalgia
- **Inflammatory Pain**
  - Arthropathies
  - Infections
  - Tissue injury
  - post-operative pain
- **Mechanical/Compressive**
  - Low back and neck pain
  - Muscuoloskeletal pain
  - Visceral pain

Pharmacological Interventions:
- **Neuropathies:**
  - Anticonvulsants (e.g. Gabapentin)
  - TCA's (e.g. Amitriptyline)
  - SNRI's (e.g. Duloxetine)
  - Topical agents (e.g. Lidocaine patch)
- **Muscle Pain:**
  - TCA's
  - Trigger point injections
- **Inflammatory Pain:**
  - NSAID's
  - Corticosteroids
  - Topical agents (e.g. Diclofenac patch)
- **Mechanical Compressive:**
  - NSAID's
  - Possible opioids

The 4 A's:
- Analgesia
- Activities of daily living
- Adverse effects
- Aberrant behavior

Non-Pharmacological Interventions:
- **Neuropathic**
  - Topical agents
  - TENs, acupuncture
  - Cognitive, behavioral therapy
  - Biofeedback, desensitization
- **Muscle Pain**
  - Modalities (hot/cold)
  - Behavioral management
  - Fitness Program
- **Inflammatory**
  - (see all pain types)
- **Mechanical, compressive pain**
  - (see all pain types)
- **All pain types:**
  - Range of motion, strengthening
  - Splinting, bracing
  - Assistive devices
  - Ergonomic modifications
  - Sleep hygiene (melatonin, TCA, Trazodone)

Opioid Selection (augmenting other treatments)
- Begin with a short-acting opioid (e.g. hydrocodone/oxycodone) while starting up; transition to a single, long-acting form (e.g. long acting morphine sulfate) when a stable daily dose is established
- When switching to a different opioid, calculate the Morphine Equivalent Dose (MED) and reduce by 25-50% initially for safety
- Avoid MED > 50-100 mg/day dose to minimize overdose risk
- Breakthrough dosing has not been shown to improve outcomes
- Avoid concurrent use of multiple opioids or co-treatment with benzodiazepines
- Avoid methadone for safety (ADR's, long variable half-life, OD risk)

NSAID – Nonsteroidal Anti-Inflammatory Drug
SNRI – Serotonin–Norepinephrine Reuptake Inhibitors
TCA   – Tricyclic Antidepressants

Suggested Readings

American Pain Society. Guideline for the use of chronic opioid therapy in chronic noncancer pain: Evidence review. 2009

Chou R, Fanciullo GJ, Fine PG, et al; American Pain Society-American Academy of Pain Medicine Opioids Guidelines Panel. Clinical guidelines for the use of chronic opioid therapy in chronic noncancer pain. J Pain 2009;10(2):113–130

Hooten W, Timming R, Belgrade M, Gaul J, Goertz M, Haake B, et al. Health care guideline: Assessment and management of chronic pain. Institute for Clinical Systems Improvement. (Updated November 2013)

Wisconsin Medical Society Task Force on Pain Management. Guidelines for the assessment and management of chronic pain. Wis Med J 2004;103(3):15

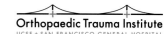
Orthopaedic Trauma Institute
UCSF + SAN FRANCISCO GENERAL HOSPITAL

Lisa Pascual, MD

Common Anticoagulant Drugs

Coumarins (vitamin K antagonists)
• Warfarin (coumadin)
Synthetic pentasaccharide inhibitors of factor Xa (low molecular weight heparins)
• Fondaparinux
• Idraparinux
• Enoxaparin
• Dalteparin

New Oral Anticoagulants (OAC)

Direct factor Xa inhibitors
• Rivaroxaban (Xarelto)
• Apixaban
Direct thrombin inhibitors
• Hirudin
• Lepirudin
• Bivalirudin
• Argatroban
• Dabigatran (Pradaxa)

Common Anti-platelet Drugs

Irreversible cyclooxygenase inhibitors
• Aspirin (ASA)
Adenosine diphosphate (ADP) receptor inhibitors
• Clopidogrel (Plavix)
• Prasugrel (Effient)
• Ticagrelor (Brilinta)

Patient-Related Risk Factors

• Increasing age
• VTE or family history of VTE
• Obesity
• Hypercoagulable state
• Congestive heart failure
• Infection
• Ventilator use
• Ascites
• Steroid use
• Alcohol use
• Pregnancy
• Oral contraception
• Hormonal replacement
• Prolonged immobility or wheelchair bound

High risk fractures/procedures for VTE

• Lower extremity fractures from the knee and above (moderate risk)
• Spinal fx with paralysis
• Polytrauma or bilateral lower extremity
• Pelvic & acetabulum fxs

Signs of Deep Vein Thrombosis (DVT)

• Calf pain
• Swelling
• Fever
• Homan's sign

Signs of Pulmonary Embolism (PE)

• Pleuritic pain
• Tachypnea
• Tachycardia
• Hypoxia

Contraindication for Chemoprophylaxis

• Brain aneurysm
• Intracranial hematoma
• Spine injury and spine surgery (controversial)
• Ongoing bleeding
• Major uncorrected coagulopathy

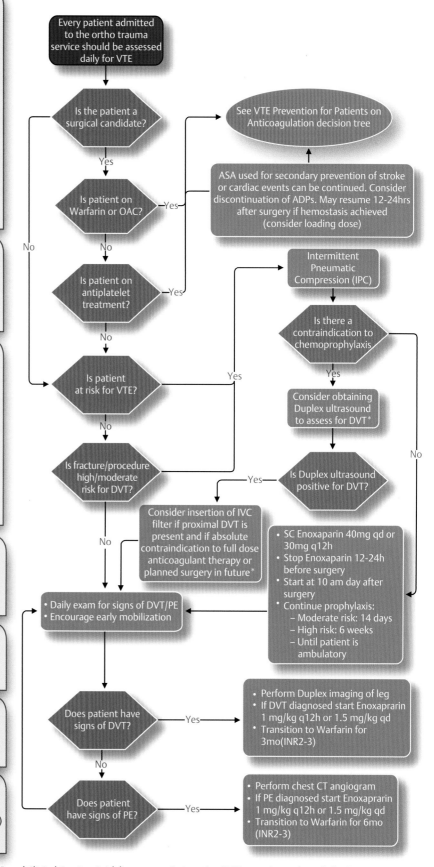

Every patient admitted to the ortho trauma service should be assessed daily for VTE

Is the patient a surgical candidate? — **No** / **Yes**

See VTE Prevention for Patients on Anticoagulation decision tree

Is patient on Warfarin or OAC? — **Yes** / **No**

ASA used for secondary prevention of stroke or cardiac events can be continued. Consider discontinuation of ADPs. May resume 12-24hrs after surgery if hemostasis achieved (consider loading dose)

Is patient on antiplatelet treatment? — **Yes** / **No**

Intermittent Pneumatic Compression (IPC)

Is patient at risk for VTE? — **Yes** / **No**

Is there a contraindication to chemoprophylaxis — **Yes** / **No**

Consider obtaining Duplex ultrasound to assess for DVT*

Is fracture/procedure high/moderate risk for DVT? — **Yes** / **No**

Is Duplex ultrasound positive for DVT?

Consider insertion of IVC filter if proximal DVT is present and if absolute contraindication to full dose anticoagulant therapy or planned surgery in future*

• SC Enoxaparin 40mg qd or 30mg q12h
• Stop Enoxaparin 12-24h before surgery
• Start at 10 am day after surgery
• Continue prophylaxis:
  – Moderate risk: 14 days
  – High risk: 6 weeks
  – Until patient is ambulatory

• Daily exam for signs of DVT/PE
• Encourage early mobilization

Does patient have signs of DVT? — **Yes** / **No**

• Perform Duplex imaging of leg
• If DVT diagnosed start Enoxaprarin 1 mg/kg q12h or 1.5 mg/kg qd
• Transition to Warfarin for 3mo(INR2-3)

Does patient have signs of PE? — **Yes**

• Perform chest CT angiogram
• If PE diagnosed start Enoxaprarin 1 mg/kg q12h or 1.5 mg/kg qd
• Transition to Warfarin for 6mo (INR2-3)

* American College of Chest Physicians Evidence-Based Clinical Practice Guidelines are against routine DVT screening and prophylactic use of inferior vena cava (IVC) filters.

Suggested Readings

Barrera, L. M., Perel, P., Ker, K., Cirocchi, R., Farinella, E., & Morales Uribe, C. H. Thrombo-prophylaxis for trauma patients. Cochrane Database of Systematic Reviews

Chassot, P., Marcucci, C., Delabays, A., & Spahn, D. (2010). Perioperative antiplatelet therapy. American Family Physician, 82(12), 1484-9.

Falck-Ytter, Y., Francis, C. W., Johanson, N. A., Curley, C., Dahl, O. E., Schulman, S., et al. (2012). Prevention of VTE in orthopedic surgery patients: Antithrombotic thera-py and prevention of thrombosis, 9th ed: American college of chest physicians ev-idence-based clinical practice guidelines. Chest, 141(2, Supplement), e278S-e325S.

Geerts, W. H., Bergqvist, D., Pineo, G. F., Heit, J. A., Samama, C. M., Lassen, M. R., et al. (2008). Prevention of venous thromboembolism: American college of chest physicians evidence-based clinical practice guidelines (8th edition). Chest, 133(6), 381S-453S.

Geerts, W. H., Pineo, G. F., Heit, J. A., Bergqvist, D., Lassen, M. R., Colwell, C. W., et al. (2004). Prevention of venous thromboembolism: The seventh ACCP conference on an-tithrombotic and thrombolytic therapy. Chest, 126(3, Supplement), 338S-400S.

NASS Evidence-Based Guideline Development Committee. (2009). Antithrombotic therapies in spine surgery North American Spine Society.

Toker, S., Hak, D., & Morgan, S. (2011). Deep vein thrombosis prophylaxis in trauma patients. Thrombosis, 505373

van Veen, J. J., & Makris, M. (2015). Management of peri-operative anti-thrombotic therapy. Anaesthesia, 70, 58-e23.

Whiting PS. (2016). Risk factors for deep venous Thrombosis following orthopaedic trauma surgery: An analysis of 56,000 patients.5(1), 2016 Jan 23;5(1):e32915. doi: 10.5812/atr.32915. eCollection 2016.

Chapter 11: VTE Prevention for Patients on Anticoagulation

Lisa Pascual, MD

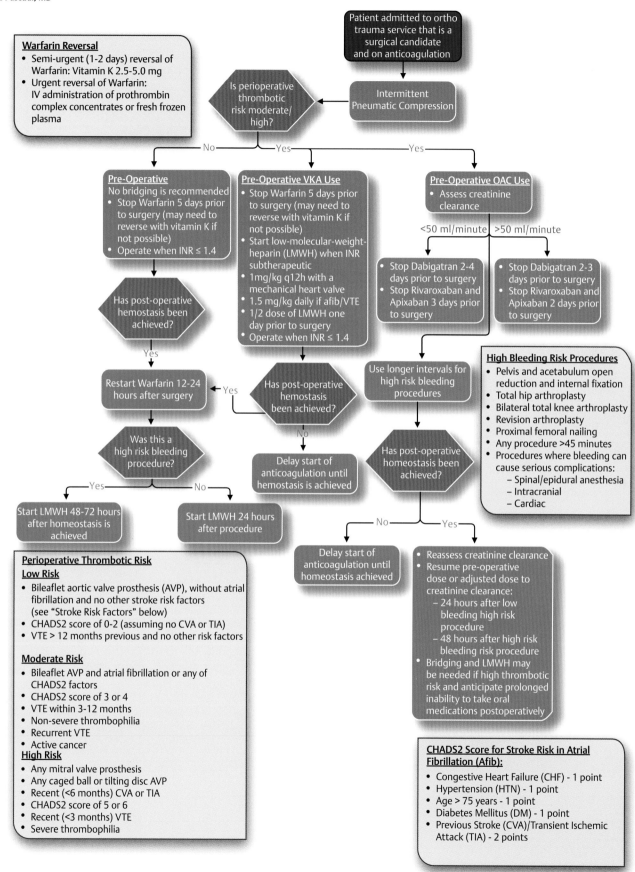

Warfarin Reversal
- Semi-urgent (1-2 days) reversal of Warfarin: Vitamin K 2.5-5.0 mg
- Urgent reversal of Warfarin: IV administration of prothrombin complex concentrates or fresh frozen plasma

Patient admitted to ortho trauma service that is a surgical candidate and on anticoagulation

Intermittent Pneumatic Compression

Is perioperative thrombotic risk moderate/ high?

No — Yes — Yes

Pre-Operative
No bridging is recommended
- Stop Warfarin 5 days prior to surgery (may need to reverse with vitamin K if not possible)
- Operate when INR ≤ 1.4

Pre-Operative VKA Use
- Stop Warfarin 5 days prior to surgery (may need to reverse with vitamin K if not possible)
- Start low-molecular-weight-heparin (LMWH) when INR subtherapeutic
- 1mg/kg q12h with a mechanical heart valve
- 1.5 mg/kg daily if afib/VTE
- 1/2 dose of LMWH one day prior to surgery
- Operate when INR ≤ 1.4

Pre-Operative OAC Use
- Assess creatinine clearance

<50 ml/minute   >50 ml/minute

- Stop Dabigatran 2-4 days prior to surgery
- Stop Rivaroxaban and Apixaban 3 days prior to surgery

- Stop Dabigatran 2-3 days prior to surgery
- Stop Rivaroxaban and Apixaban 2 days prior to surgery

Has post-operative hemostasis been achieved?

Yes

Restart Warfarin 12-24 hours after surgery

← Yes

Has post-operative hemostasis been achieved?

No

Use longer intervals for high risk bleeding procedures

Delay start of anticoagulation until hemostasis is achieved

High Bleeding Risk Procedures
- Pelvis and acetabulum open reduction and internal fixation
- Total hip arthroplasty
- Bilateral total knee arthroplasty
- Revision arthroplasty
- Proximal femoral nailing
- Any procedure >45 minutes
- Procedures where bleeding can cause serious complications:
  – Spinal/epidural anesthesia
  – Intracranial
  – Cardiac

Was this a high risk bleeding procedure?

Yes — No

Start LMWH 48-72 hours after homeostasis is achieved

Start LMWH 24 hours after procedure

Has post-operative homeostasis been achieved?

No — Yes

Delay start of anticoagulation until homeostasis achieved

- Reassess creatinine clearance
- Resume pre-operative dose or adjusted dose to creatinine clearance:
  – 24 hours after low bleeding high risk procedure
  – 48 hours after high risk bleeding risk procedure
- Bridging and LMWH may be needed if high thrombotic risk and anticipate prolonged inability to take oral medications postoperatively

Perioperative Thrombotic Risk
Low Risk
- Bileaflet aortic valve prosthesis (AVP), without atrial fibrillation and no other stroke risk factors (see "Stroke Risk Factors" below)
- CHADS2 score of 0-2 (assuming no CVA or TIA)
- VTE > 12 months previous and no other risk factors

Moderate Risk
- Bileaflet AVP and atrial fibrillation or any of CHADS2 factors
- CHADS2 score of 3 or 4
- VTE within 3-12 months
- Non-severe thrombophilia
- Recurrent VTE
- Active cancer

High Risk
- Any mitral valve prosthesis
- Any caged ball or tilting disc AVP
- Recent (<6 months) CVA or TIA
- CHADS2 score of 5 or 6
- Recent (<3 months) VTE
- Severe thrombophilia

CHADS2 Score for Stroke Risk in Atrial Fibrillation (Afib):
- Congestive Heart Failure (CHF) - 1 point
- Hypertension (HTN) - 1 point
- Age > 75 years - 1 point
- Diabetes Mellitus (DM) - 1 point
- Previous Stroke (CVA)/Transient Ischemic Attack (TIA) - 2 points

VKA – Vitamin K Antagonist (see Chapter 10)
OAC – new Oral Anti-Coagulants (see Chapter 10)

Suggested Readings

Douketis JD, Spyropoulos AC, Spencer FA, et al; American College of Chest Physicians. Perioperative management of antithrombotic therapy: Antithrombotic Therapy and Prevention of Thrombosis, 9th ed: American College of Chest Physicians Evidence-Based Clinical Practice Guidelines. Chest 2012; 141(2, Suppl):e326S–e350S

Gallego P, Apostolakis S, Lip GYH. Bridging evidence-based practice and practice-based evidence in periprocedural anticoagulation. Circulation 2012;126(13):1573–1576

van Veen JJ, Makris M. Management of peri-operative anti-thrombotic therapy. Anaesthesia 2015;70(Suppl 1):58–67, e21–e23

Chapter 12: Embolic Disease Management

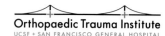

Meir T. Marmor, MD

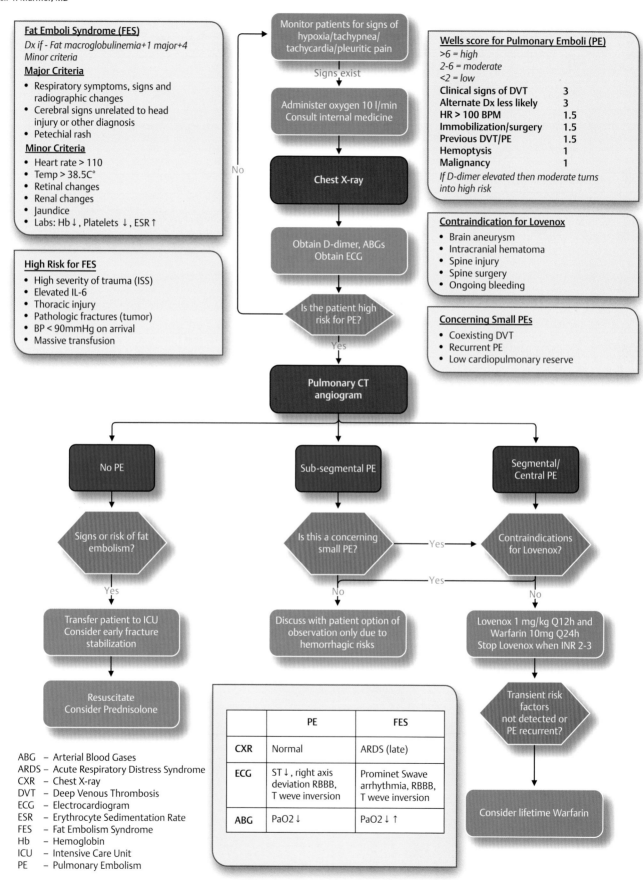

Fat Emboli Syndrome (FES)

Dx if - Fat macroglobulinemia+1 major+4 Minor criteria

Major Criteria
- Respiratory symptoms, signs and radiographic changes
- Cerebral signs unrelated to head injury or other diagnosis
- Petechial rash

Minor Criteria
- Heart rate > 110
- Temp > 38.5C°
- Retinal changes
- Renal changes
- Jaundice
- Labs: Hb↓, Platelets ↓, ESR ↑

High Risk for FES
- High severity of trauma (ISS)
- Elevated IL-6
- Thoracic injury
- Pathologic fractures (tumor)
- BP < 90mmHg on arrival
- Massive transfusion

Monitor patients for signs of hypoxia/tachypnea/tachycardia/pleuritic pain

Signs exist

Administer oxygen 10 l/min Consult internal medicine

Chest X-ray

Obtain D-dimer, ABGs Obtain ECG

Is the patient high risk for PE?

No

Yes

Pulmonary CT angiogram

Wells score for Pulmonary Emboli (PE)

>6 = high
2-6 = moderate
<2 = low

Clinical signs of DVT	3
Alternate Dx less likely	3
HR > 100 BPM	1.5
Immobilization/surgery	1.5
Previous DVT/PE	1.5
Hemoptysis	1
Malignancy	1

If D-dimer elevated then moderate turns into high risk

Contraindication for Lovenox
- Brain aneurysm
- Intracranial hematoma
- Spine injury
- Spine surgery
- Ongoing bleeding

Concerning Small PEs
- Coexisting DVT
- Recurrent PE
- Low cardiopulmonary reserve

No PE

Signs or risk of fat embolism?

Yes

Transfer patient to ICU Consider early fracture stabilization

Resuscitate Consider Prednisolone

Sub-segmental PE

Is this a concerning small PE?

Yes

No

Discuss with patient option of observation only due to hemorrhagic risks

Segmental/ Central PE

Contraindications for Lovenox?

Yes

No

Lovenox 1 mg/kg Q12h and Warfarin 10mg Q24h Stop Lovenox when INR 2-3

Transient risk factors not detected or PE recurrent?

Consider lifetime Warfarin

	PE	FES
CXR	Normal	ARDS (late)
ECG	ST ↓, right axis deviation RBBB, T weve inversion	Prominet Swave arrhythmia, RBBB, T weve inversion
ABG	PaO2 ↓	PaO2 ↓ ↑

ABG – Arterial Blood Gases
ARDS – Acute Respiratory Distress Syndrome
CXR – Chest X-ray
DVT – Deep Venous Thrombosis
ECG – Electrocardiogram
ESR – Erythrocyte Sedimentation Rate
FES – Fat Embolism Syndrome
Hb   – Hemoglobin
ICU – Intensive Care Unit
PE   – Pulmonary Embolism

Suggested Readings

Wells PS, Anderson DR, Rodger M, et al. Derivation of a simple clinical model to categorize patients probability of pulmonary embolism: increasing the models utility with the SimpliRED D-dimer. Thromb Haemost 2000;83(3):416–420

Goodman LR. Small pulmonary emboli: what do we know? Radiology 2005;234 (3):654–658

Gurd AR, Wilson RI. The fat embolism syndrome. J Bone Joint Surg Br 1974;56B(3): 408–416

White T, Petrisor BA, Bhandari M. Prevention of fat embolism syndrome. Injury 2006;37(Suppl 4):S59–S67 Review

Chapter 13: Heterotopic Ossification (HO)

Harry Jergesen, MD

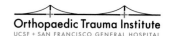

Risk for HO

- Brain Injury
- Prior history of HO
- Family history of HO
- Existing HO
- Extensive hip surgery
- Polytrauma patient
- Spinal cord injury
- Ankylosing Spondylitis
- Diffuse Idiopathic Skeletal Hyperostosis (DISH)

Prophylactic Therapy

NSAIDS
- Indomethacin 75mg/day for 10-42 days

Radiation
- 700cGy <4 hours before surgery or within 72 hours after surgery

HO Signs, Symptoms and Complications

- Erythema
- Swelling
- Warmth
- Reduced range of motion
- Neurovascular compromise
- Severe pain

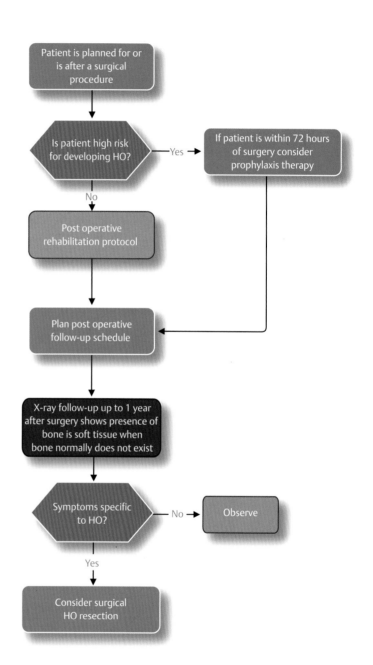

Suggested Readings

Board TN, Karva A, Board RE, Gambhir AK, Porter ML. The prophylaxis and treatment of heterotopic ossification following lower limb arthroplasty. J Bone Joint Surg Br 2007;89(4):434–440

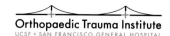
Meir T. Marmor, MD

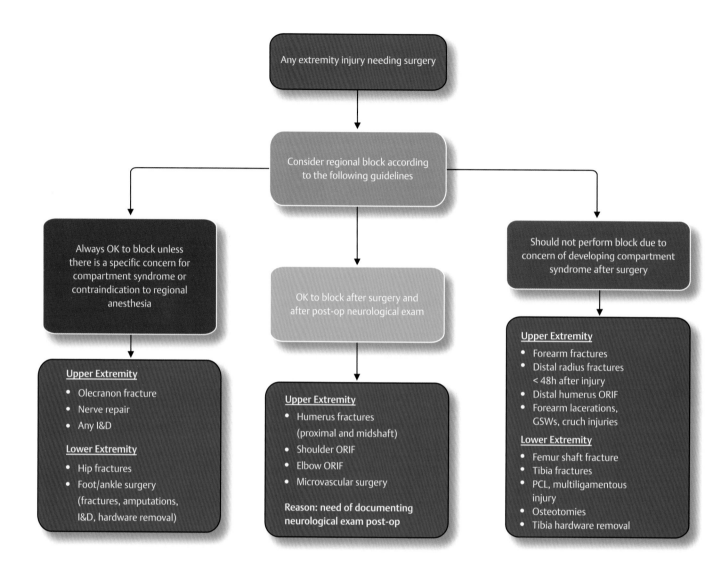

Any extremity injury needing surgery

Consider regional block according to the following guidelines

Always OK to block unless there is a specific concern for compartment syndrome or contraindication to regional anesthesia

OK to block after surgery and after post-op neurological exam

Should not perform block due to concern of developing compartment syndrome after surgery

<u>**Upper Extremity**</u>
- Olecranon fracture
- Nerve repair
- Any I&D

<u>**Lower Extremity**</u>
- Hip fractures
- Foot/ankle surgery (fractures, amputations, I&D, hardware removal)

<u>**Upper Extremity**</u>
- Humerus fractures (proximal and midshaft)
- Shoulder ORIF
- Elbow ORIF
- Microvascular surgery

Reason: need of documenting neurological exam post-op

<u>**Upper Extremity**</u>
- Forearm fractures
- Distal radius fractures < 48h after injury
- Distal humerus ORIF
- Forearm lacerations, GSWs, cruch injuries

<u>**Lower Extremity**</u>
- Femur shaft fracture
- Tibia fractures
- PCL, multiligamentous injury
- Osteotomies
- Tibia hardware removal

<u>**Contraindications for Regional Anesthesia:**</u>
- Maximal anesthetic dose has been exceeded
- Infection at the injection site
- An allergy to local anesthetics
- Preexisting neuropathology

<u>**Relative Contraindications:**</u>
- Dementia
- Child
- Bleeding disorder

GSW – Gun Shot Wound
I&D – Irrigation and Debridement
ORIF – Open Reduction Internal Fixation
PCL – Posterior Cruciate Ligament

Suggested Readings

Bruce BG, Green A, Blaine TA, Wesner LV. Brachial plexus blocks for upper extremity orthopaedic surgery. *J Am Acad Orthop Surg.* Jan 2012;20(1):38-47.

Wu CL, Rouse LM, Chen JM, Miller RJ. Comparison of postoperative pain in patients receiving interscalene block or general anesthesia for shoulder surgery. *Orthopedics.* Jan 2002;25(1):45-48.

Chapter 15: Traumatic Anterior Shoulder Instability

Nicolas Lee, MD

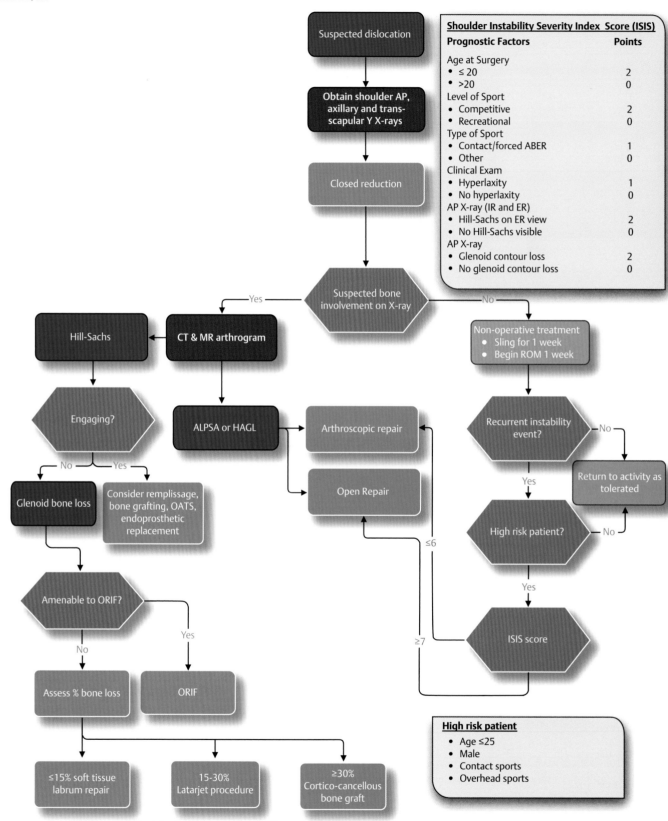

Shoulder Instability Severity Index Score (ISIS)

Prognostic Factors	Points
Age at Surgery	
• ≤ 20	2
• >20	0
Level of Sport	
• Competitive	2
• Recreational	0
Type of Sport	
• Contact/forced ABER	1
• Other	0
Clinical Exam	
• Hyperlaxity	1
• No hyperlaxity	0
AP X-ray (IR and ER)	
• Hill-Sachs on ER view	2
• No Hill-Sachs visible	0
AP X-ray	
• Glenoid contour loss	2
• No glenoid contour loss	0

Flowchart:

- Suspected dislocation →
- Obtain shoulder AP, axillary and trans-scapular Y X-rays →
- Closed reduction →
- Suspected bone involvement on X-ray
  - Yes → CT & MR arthrogram
    - Hill-Sachs
      - Engaging?
        - No → Glenoid bone loss → Amenable to ORIF?
          - No → Assess % bone loss
            - ≤15% soft tissue labrum repair
            - 15-30% Latarjet procedure
            - ≥30% Cortico-cancellous bone graft
          - Yes → ORIF
        - Yes → Consider remplissage, bone grafting, OATS, endoprosthetic replacement
    - ALPSA or HAGL → Arthroscopic repair / Open Repair
  - No → Non-operative treatment
    - Sling for 1 week
    - Begin ROM 1 week
    - → Recurrent instability event?
      - No → Return to activity as tolerated
      - Yes → High risk patient?
        - No → Return to activity as tolerated
        - Yes → ISIS score
          - ≤6 → Arthroscopic repair
          - ≥7 → Open Repair

High risk patient
- Age ≤25
- Male
- Contact sports
- Overhead sports

ALPSA – Anterior Labroligamentous Periosteal Sleeve Avulsion
HAGL – Humeral Avulsion of the Glenohumeral Ligament
ABER – Abduction External Rotation
OATS – Osteochondral Autograft Transfer System
IR – Internal Rotation
ER – External Rotation

Suggested Readings

Balg F, Boileau P. The instability severity index score. A simple pre-operative score to select patients for arthroscopic or open shoulder stabilisation. J Bone Joint Surg Br 2007;89(11):1470–1477

Allain J, Goutallier D, Glorion C. Long-term results of the Latarjet procedure for the treatment of anterior instability of the shoulder. J Bone Joint Surg Am 1998;80(6):841–852

Øster A. Recurrent anterior dislocation of the shoulder treated by the Eden-Hybinette operation. Follow-up on 78 cases. Acta Orthop Scand 1969;40(1):43–52

Meir T. Marmor, MD

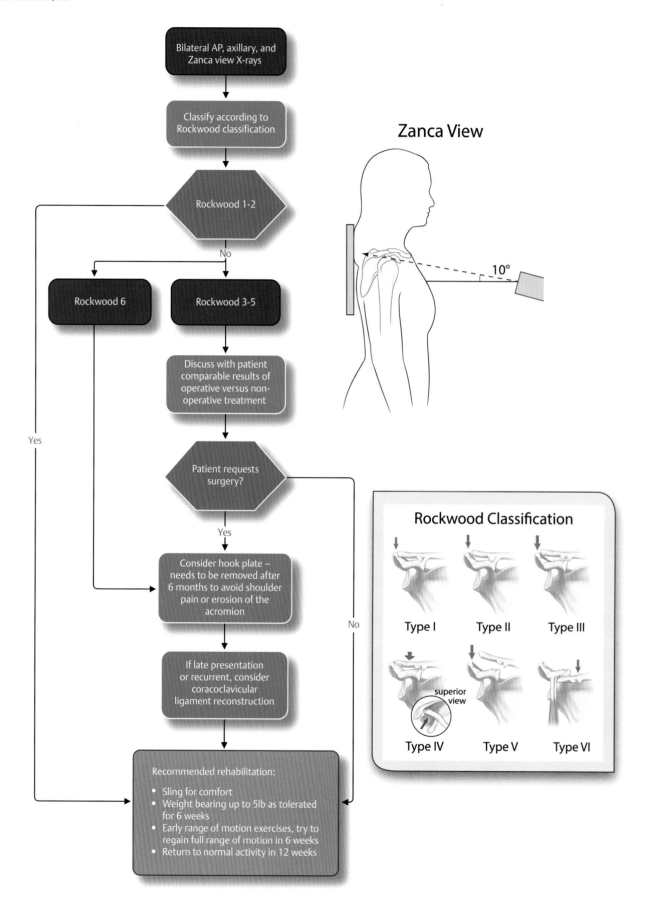

Bilateral AP, axillary, and Zanca view X-rays

Classify according to Rockwood classification

Rockwood 1-2

No

Rockwood 6

Rockwood 3-5

Yes

Discuss with patient comparable results of operative versus non-operative treatment

Patient requests surgery?

Yes

No

Consider hook plate – needs to be removed after 6 months to avoid shoulder pain or erosion of the acromion

If late presentation or recurrent, consider coracoclavicular ligament reconstruction

Recommended rehabilitation:

- Sling for comfort
- Weight bearing up to 5lb as tolerated for 6 weeks
- Early range of motion exercises, try to regain full range of motion in 6 weeks
- Return to normal activity in 12 weeks

Zanca View

10°

Rockwood Classification

Type I Type II Type III

Type IV superior view Type V Type VI

Suggested Readings

Canadian Orthopaedic Trauma Society. Multicenter Randomized Clinical Trial of Non-operative Versus Operative Treatment of Acute Acromio-Clavicular Joint Dislocation. J Orthop Trauma 2015;29(11):479–487

Chapter 17: Sternoclavicular Dislocation (SCD)

Utku Kandemir, MD

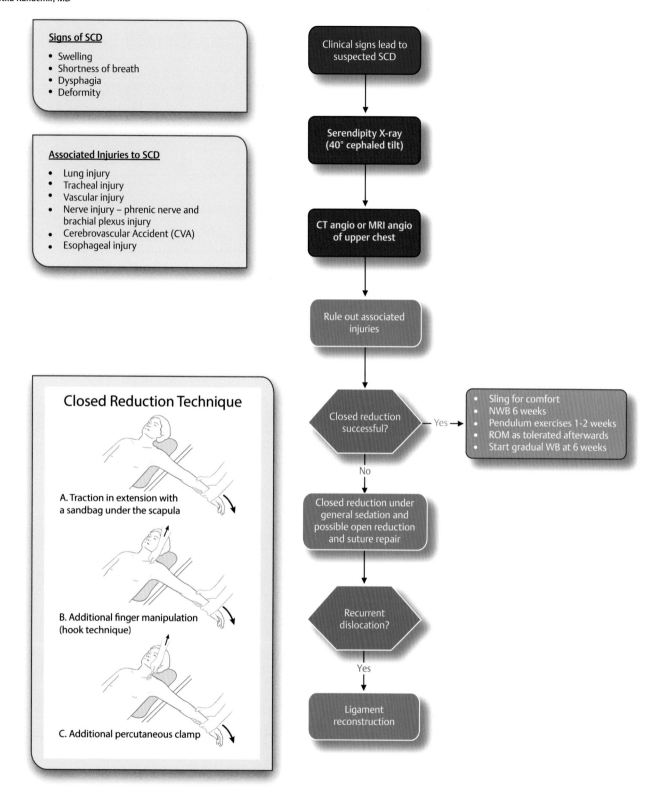

Signs of SCD

- Swelling
- Shortness of breath
- Dysphagia
- Deformity

Associated Injuries to SCD

- Lung injury
- Tracheal injury
- Vascular injury
- Nerve injury – phrenic nerve and brachial plexus injury
- Cerebrovascular Accident (CVA)
- Esophageal injury

Closed Reduction Technique

A. Traction in extension with a sandbag under the scapula

B. Additional finger manipulation (hook technique)

C. Additional percutaneous clamp

Clinical signs lead to suspected SCD

↓

Serendipity X-ray (40° cephaled tilt)

↓

CT angio or MRI angio of upper chest

↓

Rule out associated injuries

↓

Closed reduction successful? —Yes→
- Sling for comfort
- NWB 6 weeks
- Pendulum exercises 1-2 weeks
- ROM as tolerated afterwards
- Start gradual WB at 6 weeks

No ↓

Closed reduction under general sedation and possible open reduction and suture repair

↓

Recurrent dislocation?

Yes ↓

Ligament reconstruction

NWB – Non Weight Bearing
ROM – Range Of Motion
WB – Weight Bearing

Suggested Readings

Eskola A, Vainionpää S, Vastamäki M, Slätis P, Rokkanen P. Operation for old sternocla-vicular dislocation. Results in 12 cases. J Bone Joint Surg Br 1989;71(1):63–65

Chapter 18: Clavicle Fractures

Paul Toogood, MD

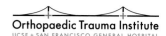

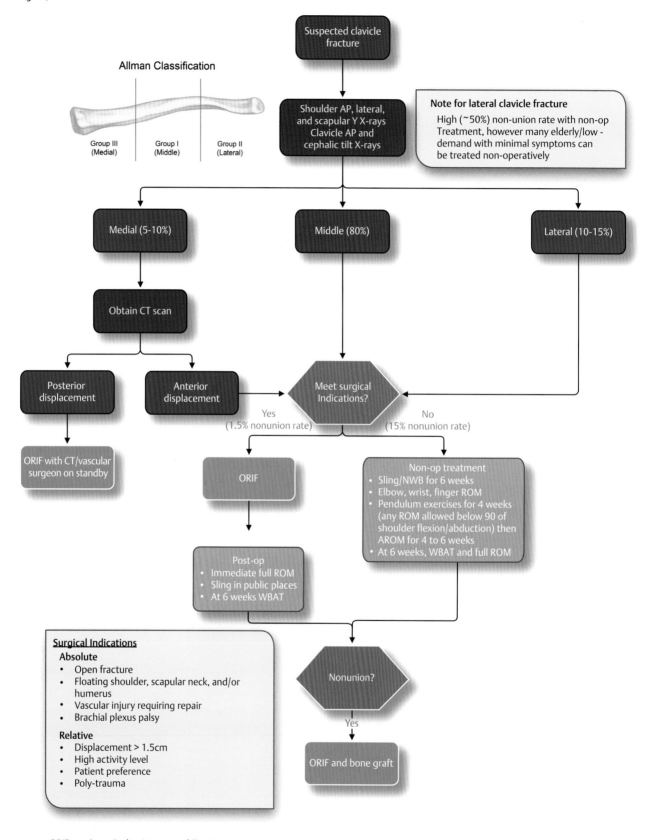

Allman Classification

Group III (Medial) | Group I (Middle) | Group II (Lateral)

Suspected clavicle fracture

Shoulder AP, lateral, and scapular Y X-rays
Clavicle AP and cephalic tilt X-rays

Note for lateral clavicle fracture
High (~50%) non-union rate with non-op Treatment, however many elderly/low-demand with minimal symptoms can be treated non-operatively

Medial (5-10%) | Middle (80%) | Lateral (10-15%)

Obtain CT scan

Posterior displacement | Anterior displacement

Meet surgical Indications?

Yes (1.5% nonunion rate) | No (15% nonunion rate)

ORIF with CT/vascular surgeon on standby

ORIF

Non-op treatment
- Sling/NWB for 6 weeks
- Elbow, wrist, finger ROM
- Pendulum exercises for 4 weeks (any ROM allowed below 90 of shoulder flexion/abduction) then AROM for 4 to 6 weeks
- At 6 weeks, WBAT and full ROM

Post-op
- Immediate full ROM
- Sling in public places
- At 6 weeks WBAT

Surgical Indications
Absolute
- Open fracture
- Floating shoulder, scapular neck, and/or humerus
- Vascular injury requiring repair
- Brachial plexus palsy

Relative
- Displacement > 1.5cm
- High activity level
- Patient preference
- Poly-trauma

Nonunion?

Yes

ORIF and bone graft

ORIF   – Open Reduction Internal Fixation
ROM   – Range Of Motion
WBAT – Weight Bearing As Tolerated
NWB   – Non Weight Bearing

Suggested Readings

McKee RC, Whelan DB, Schemitsch EH, McKee MD. Operative versus nonoperative care of displaced midshaft clavicular fractures: a meta-analysis of randomized clinical trials. J Bone Joint Surg Am 2012;94(8):675–684

Khan LA, Bradnock TJ, Scott C, Robinson CM. Fractures of the clavicle. J Bone Joint Surg Am 2009;91(2):447–460

Chapter 19: Scapulothoracic Dissociation (STD)

Utku Kandemir, MD

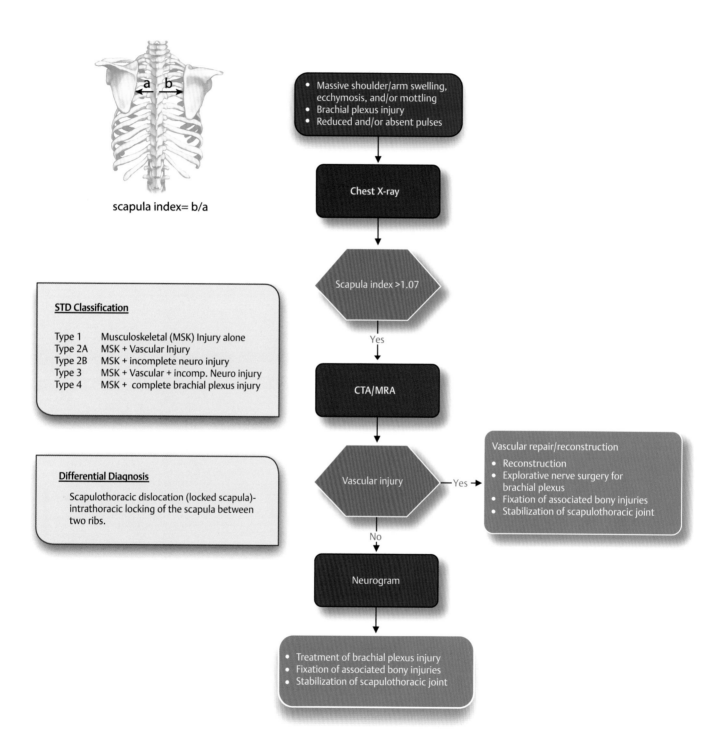

scapula index= b/a

STD Classification

Type 1	Musculoskeletal (MSK) Injury alone
Type 2A	MSK + Vascular Injury
Type 2B	MSK + incomplete neuro injury
Type 3	MSK + Vascular + incomp. Neuro injury
Type 4	MSK + complete brachial plexus injury

Differential Diagnosis

Scapulothoracic dislocation (locked scapula)- intrathoracic locking of the scapula between two ribs.

- Massive shoulder/arm swelling, ecchymosis, and/or mottling
- Brachial plexus injury
- Reduced and/or absent pulses

Chest X-ray

Scapula index >1.07

Yes

CTA/MRA

Vascular injury → Yes →

Vascular repair/reconstruction
- Reconstruction
- Explorative nerve surgery for brachial plexus
- Fixation of associated bony injuries
- Stabilization of scapulothoracic joint

No

Neurogram

- Treatment of brachial plexus injury
- Fixation of associated bony injuries
- Stabilization of scapulothoracic joint

Suggested Readings

Zelle BA, Pape HC, Gerich TG, Garapati R, Ceylan B, Krettek C. Functional outcome following scapulothoracic dissociation. J Bone Joint Surg Am 2004;86-A(1):2–8

Hollinshead R, James KW. Scapulothoracic dislocation (locked scapula). A case report. J Bone Joint Surg Am 1979;61(7):1102–1103

Oreck SL, Burgess A, Levine AM. Traumatic lateral displacement of the scapula: a radiographic sign of neurovascular disruption. J Bone Joint Surg Am 1984;66(5):758–763

Chapter 20: Scapula Fractures

Utku Kandemir, MD

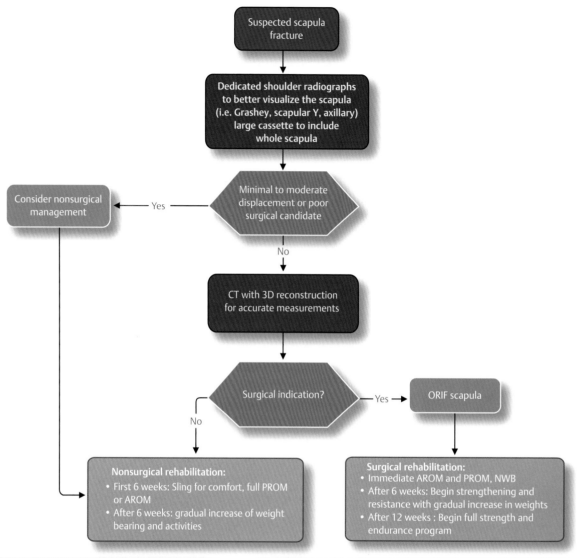

Suspected scapula fracture

↓

Dedicated shoulder radiographs to better visualize the scapula (i.e. Grashey, scapular Y, axillary) large cassette to include whole scapula

↓

Minimal to moderate displacement or poor surgical candidate — Yes → **Consider nonsurgical management**

↓ No

CT with 3D reconstruction for accurate measurements

↓

Surgical indication? — Yes → **ORIF scapula**

↓ No

Nonsurgical rehabilitation:
- First 6 weeks: Sling for comfort, full PROM or AROM
- After 6 weeks: gradual increase of weight bearing and activities

Surgical rehabilitation:
- Immediate AROM and PROM, NWB
- After 6 weeks: Begin strengthening and resistance with gradual increase in weights
- After 12 weeks : Begin full strength and endurance program

Surgical Indications and Measurement Techniques

Intra-articular gap/step-off
Relative: ≥3 – 10 mm

Relative: 20% – 30% glenoid involvement

Medialization
Relative: ≥10 – 20mm

Glenopolar angle
Relative: ≤20° – 22°

Angulation
Relative: ≥30° – 45°

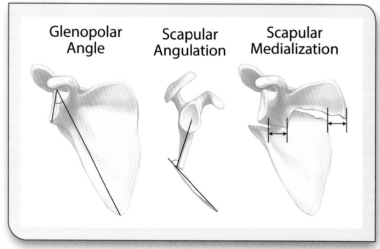

Glenopolar Angle   Scapular Angulation   Scapular Medialization

---

AROM – Active Range Of Motion
PROM – Passive Range Of Motion
ROM – Range Of Motion

Suggested Readings

Cole PA, Gauger EM, Schroder LK. Management of scapular fractures. J Am Acad Orthop Surg 2012;20(3):130–141

Chapter 21: Proximal Humerus Fractures

Utku Kandemir, MD

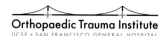

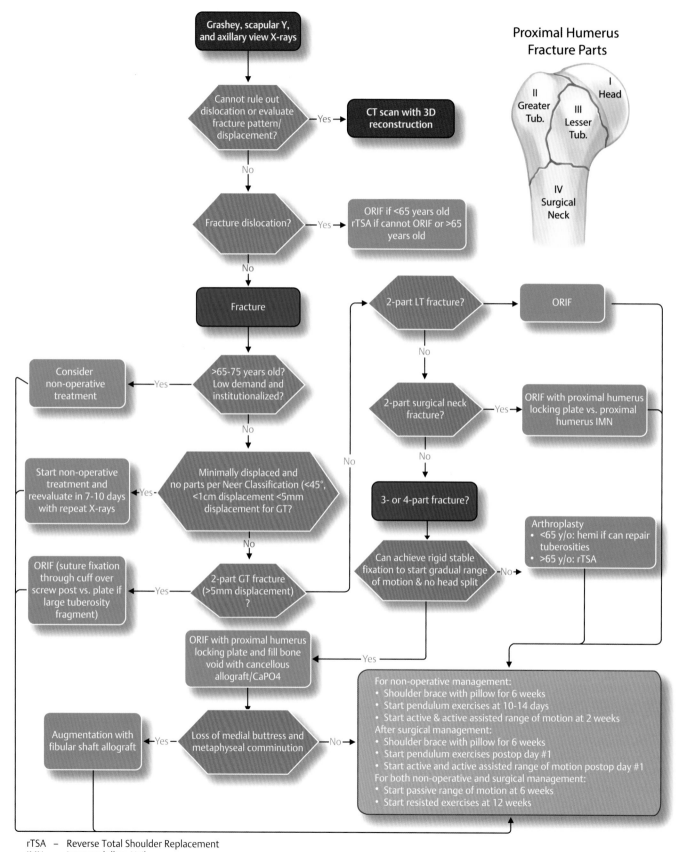

Proximal Humerus Fracture Parts

I Head
II Greater Tub.
III Lesser Tub.
IV Surgical Neck

Grashey, scapular Y, and axillary view X-rays

Cannot rule out dislocation or evaluate fracture pattern/displacement? — Yes → **CT scan with 3D reconstruction**

No ↓

Fracture dislocation? — Yes → ORIF if <65 years old rTSA if cannot ORIF or >65 years old

No ↓

Fracture

>65-75 years old? Low demand and institutionalized? — Yes → Consider non-operative treatment

No ↓

Minimally displaced and no parts per Neer Classification (<45°, <1cm displacement <5mm displacement for GT? — Yes → Start non-operative treatment and reevaluate in 7-10 days with repeat X-rays

No ↓

2-part GT fracture (>5mm displacement)? — Yes → ORIF (suture fixation through cuff over screw post vs. plate if large tuberosity fragment)

ORIF with proximal humerus locking plate and fill bone void with cancellous allograft/CaPO4

Loss of medial buttress and metaphyseal comminution — Yes → Augmentation with fibular shaft allograft

2-part LT fracture? — Yes → ORIF

No ↓

2-part surgical neck fracture? — Yes → ORIF with proximal humerus locking plate vs. proximal humerus IMN

No ↓

3- or 4-part fracture?

Can achieve rigid stable fixation to start gradual range of motion & no head split — No → Arthroplasty
• <65 y/o: hemi if can repair tuberosities
• >65 y/o: rTSA

Yes ↓

For non-operative management:
• Shoulder brace with pillow for 6 weeks
• Start pendulum exercises at 10-14 days
• Start active & active assisted range of motion at 2 weeks
After surgical management:
• Shoulder brace with pillow for 6 weeks
• Start pendulum exercises postop day #1
• Start active and active assisted range of motion postop day #1
For both non-operative and surgical management:
• Start passive range of motion at 6 weeks
• Start resisted exercises at 12 weeks

rTSA – Reverse Total Shoulder Replacement
IMN – Intramedullary Nail
ORIF – Open Reduction Internal Fixation

Suggested Readings

Neer CS II. Displaced proximal humeral fractures. I. Classification and evaluation. J Bone Joint Surg Am 1970;52(6):1077–1089

Chapter 22: Humeral Shaft Fractures

Paul Toogood, MD

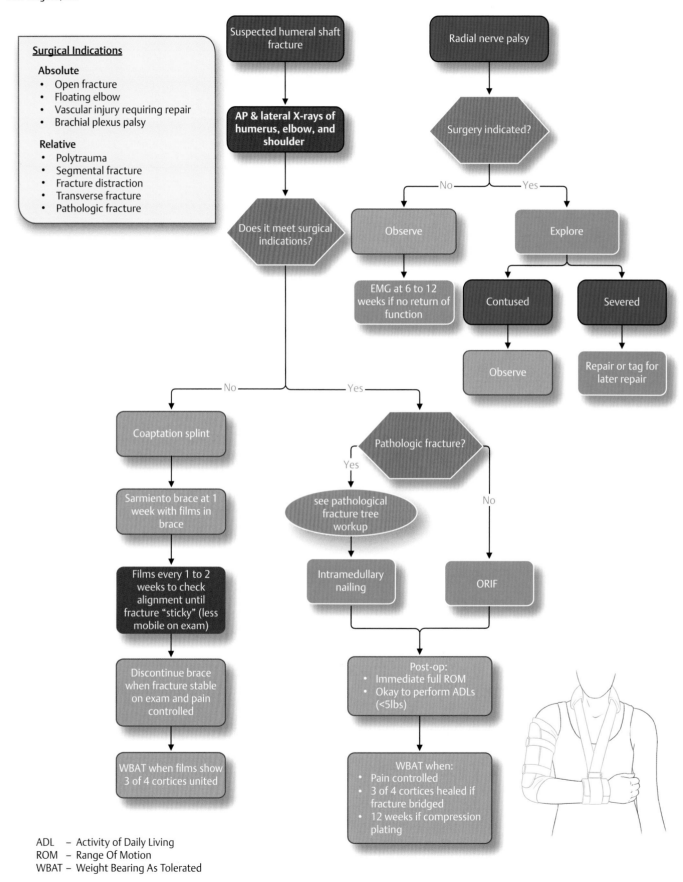

Surgical Indications

Absolute
- Open fracture
- Floating elbow
- Vascular injury requiring repair
- Brachial plexus palsy

Relative
- Polytrauma
- Segmental fracture
- Fracture distraction
- Transverse fracture
- Pathologic fracture

Suspected humeral shaft fracture

AP & lateral X-rays of humerus, elbow, and shoulder

Does it meet surgical indications?

Radial nerve palsy

Surgery indicated?

No — Observe → EMG at 6 to 12 weeks if no return of function

Yes — Explore → Contused → Observe; Severed → Repair or tag for later repair

No — Coaptation splint → Sarmiento brace at 1 week with films in brace → Films every 1 to 2 weeks to check alignment until fracture "sticky" (less mobile on exam) → Discontinue brace when fracture stable on exam and pain controlled → WBAT when films show 3 of 4 cortices united

Yes — Pathologic fracture?
- Yes → see pathological fracture tree workup → Intramedullary nailing
- No → ORIF

Post-op:
- Immediate full ROM
- Okay to perform ADLs (<5lbs)

WBAT when:
- Pain controlled
- 3 of 4 cortices healed if fracture bridged
- 12 weeks if compression plating

ADL – Activity of Daily Living
ROM – Range Of Motion
WBAT – Weight Bearing As Tolerated

Suggested Readings

Sarmiento A, Kinman PB, Galvin EG, Schmitt RH, Phillips JG. Functional bracing of fractures of the shaft of the humerus. J Bone Joint Surg Am 1977;59(5):596–601

Wang X, Chen Z, Shao Y, Ma Y, Fu D, Xia Q. A meta-analysis of plate fixation versus intramedullary nailing for humeral shaft fractures. J Orthop Sci 2013;18(3):388–397

Sarahrudi K, Wolf H, Funovics P, Pajenda G, Hausmann JT, Vécsei V. Surgical treatment of pathological fractures of the shaft of the humerus. J Trauma 2009;66(3):789–794

Paul Toogood, MD

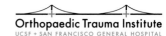

Orthopaedic Trauma Institute
UCSF + SAN FRANCISCO GENERAL HOSPITAL

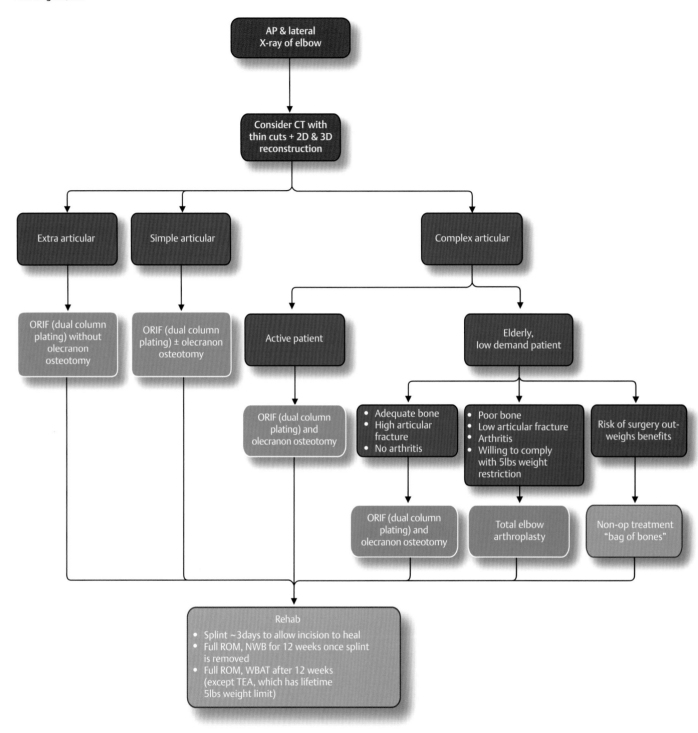

AP & lateral
X-ray of elbow

Consider CT with
thin cuts + 2D & 3D
reconstruction

Extra articular

Simple articular

Complex articular

ORIF (dual column
plating) without
olecranon
osteotomy

ORIF (dual column
plating) ± olecranon
osteotomy

Active patient

Elderly,
low demand patient

ORIF (dual column
plating) and
olecranon osteotomy

- Adequate bone
- High articular fracture
- No arthritis

- Poor bone
- Low articular fracture
- Arthritis
- Willing to comply with 5lbs weight restriction

Risk of surgery out-weighs benefits

ORIF (dual column
plating) and
olecranon osteotomy

Total elbow
arthroplasty

Non-op treatment
"bag of bones"

Rehab
- Splint ~3days to allow incision to heal
- Full ROM, NWB for 12 weeks once splint is removed
- Full ROM, WBAT after 12 weeks (except TEA, which has lifetime 5lbs weight limit)

AP   – Anterior Posterior
NWB   – Non Weight Bearing
ORIF – Open Reduction Internal Fixation
ROM   – Range Of Motion
TEA   – Total Elbow Arthroplasty
WBAT – Weight Bearing As Tolerated

Suggested Readings

McKee MD, Veillette CJ, Hall JA, et al. A multicenter, prospective, randomized, controlled trial of open reduction--internal fixation versus total elbow arthroplasty for displaced intra-articular distal humeral fractures in elderly patients. J Shoulder Elbow Surg 2009;18(1):3–12

Caravaggi P, Laratta JL, Yoon RS, et al. Internal fixation of the distal humerus: a comprehensive biomechanical study evaluating current fixation techniques. J Orthop Trauma 2014;28(4):222–226

Utku Kandemir, MD

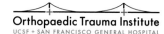
Orthopaedic Trauma Institute
UCSF + SAN FRANCISCO GENERAL HOSPITAL

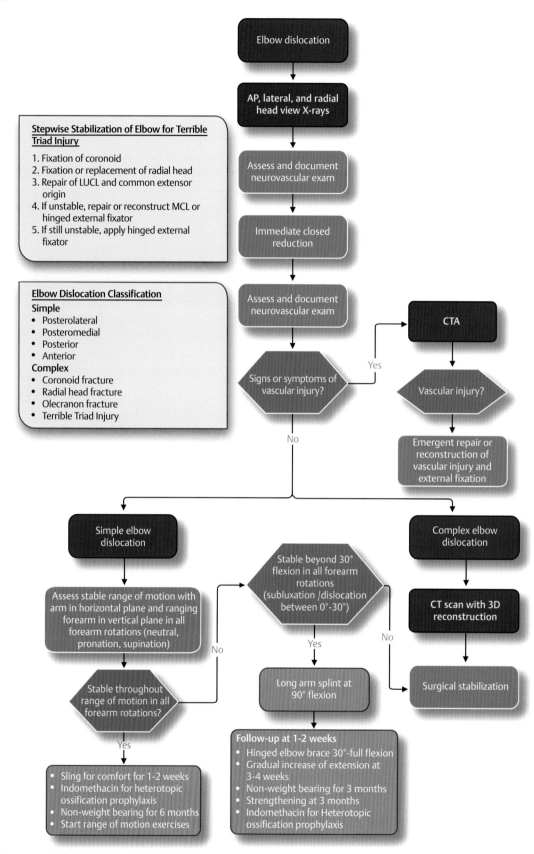

Stepwise Stabilization of Elbow for Terrible Triad Injury

1. Fixation of coronoid
2. Fixation or replacement of radial head
3. Repair of LUCL and common extensor origin
4. If unstable, repair or reconstruct MCL or hinged external fixator
5. If still unstable, apply hinged external fixator

Elbow Dislocation Classification

Simple
- Posterolateral
- Posteromedial
- Posterior
- Anterior

Complex
- Coronoid fracture
- Radial head fracture
- Olecranon fracture
- Terrible Triad Injury

Elbow dislocation

↓

AP, lateral, and radial head view X-rays

↓

Assess and document neurovascular exam

↓

Immediate closed reduction

↓

Assess and document neurovascular exam

↓

Signs or symptoms of vascular injury? — Yes → CTA → Vascular injury? → Emergent repair or reconstruction of vascular injury and external fixation

No ↓

Simple elbow dislocation

↓

Assess stable range of motion with arm in horizontal plane and ranging forearm in vertical plane in all forearm rotations (neutral, pronation, supination)

↓

Stable throughout range of motion in all forearm rotations?

No → Stable beyond 30° flexion in all forearm rotations (subluxation /dislocation between 0°-30°)

Yes ↓ → Long arm splint at 90° flexion

Follow-up at 1-2 weeks
- Hinged elbow brace 30°-full flexion
- Gradual increase of extension at 3-4 weeks
- Non-weight bearing for 3 months
- Strengthening at 3 months
- Indomethacin for Heterotopic ossification prophylaxis

Yes ↓

- Sling for comfort for 1-2 weeks
- Indomethacin for heterotopic ossification prophylaxis
- Non-weight bearing for 6 months
- Start range of motion exercises

Complex elbow dislocation

↓

CT scan with 3D reconstruction

↓

No → Surgical stabilization

LUCL – Lateral Ulnar Collateral Ligament
MCL – Medial Collateral Ligament

Suggested Readings

Pugh DM, Wild LM, Schemitsch EH, King GJ, McKee MD. Standard surgical protocol to treat elbow dislocations with radial head and coronoid fractures. J Bone Joint Surg Am 2004;86-A(6):1122–1130

Chapter 25: Radial Head Fractures

Nicolas Lee, MD

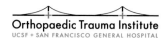
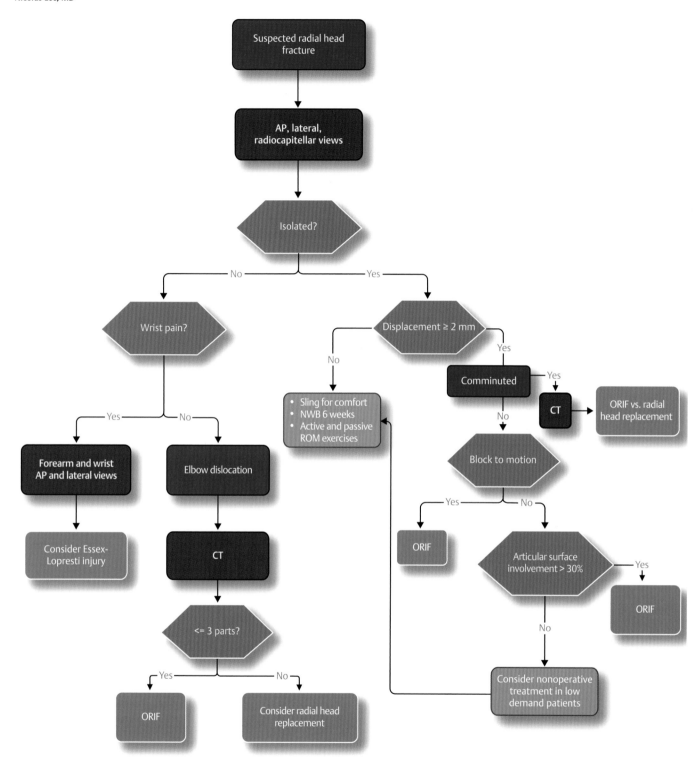

NWB – Non Weight Bearing
ORIF – Open Reduction Internal Fixation
ROM – Range Of Motion

Suggested Readings

Yoon A, Athwal GS, Faber KJ, King GJ. Radial head fractures. J Hand Surg Am 2012;37(12):2626–2634

Tejwani NC, Mehta H. Fractures of the radial head and neck: current concepts in management. J Am Acad Orthop Surg 2007;15(7):380–387

Chapter 26: Capitellum Fractures

Utku Kandemir, MD

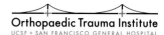

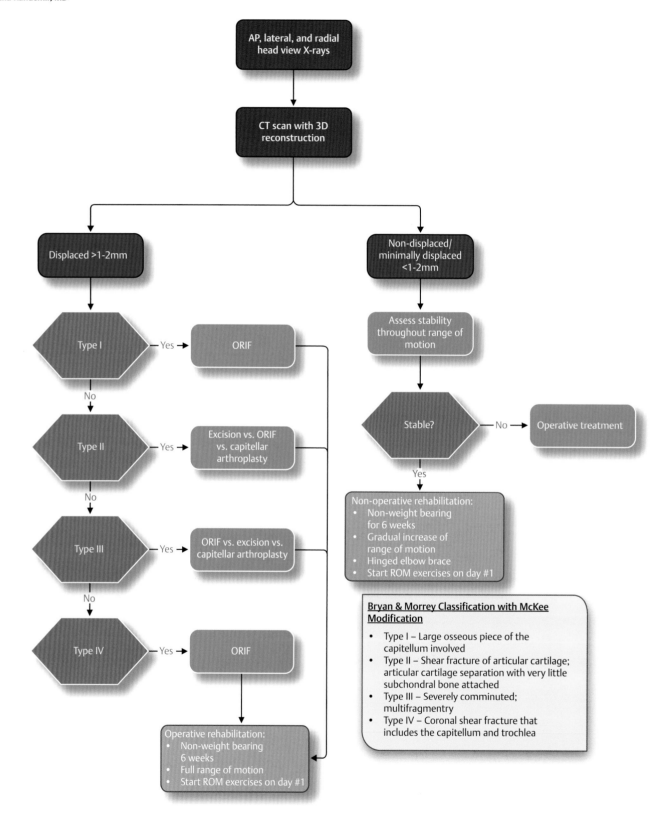

AP, lateral, and radial head view X-rays

↓

CT scan with 3D reconstruction

Displaced >1-2mm

Non-displaced/ minimally displaced <1-2mm

Type I — Yes → ORIF

No ↓

Type II — Yes → Excision vs. ORIF vs. capitellar arthroplasty

No ↓

Type III — Yes → ORIF vs. excision vs. capitellar arthroplasty

No ↓

Type IV — Yes → ORIF

Assess stability throughout range of motion

↓

Stable? — No → Operative treatment

Yes ↓

Non-operative rehabilitation:
- Non-weight bearing for 6 weeks
- Gradual increase of range of motion
- Hinged elbow brace
- Start ROM exercises on day #1

Bryan & Morrey Classification with McKee Modification

- Type I – Large osseous piece of the capitellum involved
- Type II – Shear fracture of articular cartilage; articular cartilage separation with very little subchondral bone attached
- Type III – Severely comminuted; multifragmentry
- Type IV – Coronal shear fracture that includes the capitellum and trochlea

Operative rehabilitation:
- Non-weight bearing 6 weeks
- Full range of motion
- Start ROM exercises on day #1

AP   – Anterior to Posterior
ORIF – Open Reduction Internal Fixation
ROM – Range Of Motion

Suggested Readings

McKee MD, Jupiter JB, Bamberger HB. Coronal shear fractures of the distal end of the humerus. J Bone Joint Surg Am 1996;78(1):49–54

Chapter 27: Olecranon Fractures

Nicolas Lee, MD

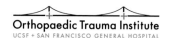
Orthopaedic Trauma Institute
UCSF + SAN FRANCISCO GENERAL HOSPITAL

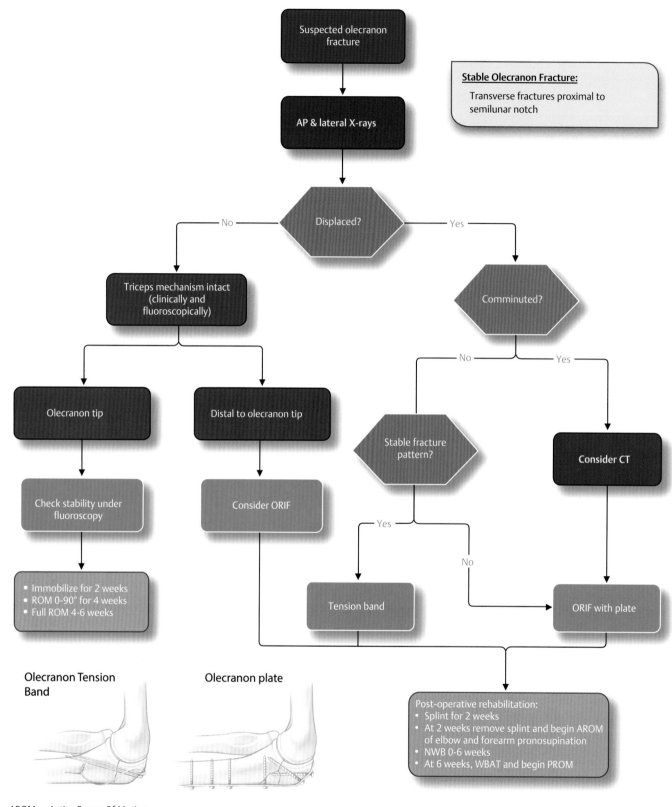

Stable Olecranon Fracture:
Transverse fractures proximal to semilunar notch

Suspected olecranon fracture

AP & lateral X-rays

Displaced?

No → Triceps mechanism intact (clinically and fluoroscopically)

Yes → Comminuted?

Olecranon tip

Distal to olecranon tip

Check stability under fluoroscopy

Consider ORIF

- Immobilize for 2 weeks
- ROM 0-90° for 4 weeks
- Full ROM 4-6 weeks

Comminuted? No → Stable fracture pattern?

Comminuted? Yes → Consider CT

Stable fracture pattern? Yes → Tension band

Stable fracture pattern? No → ORIF with plate

Post-operative rehabilitation:
- Splint for 2 weeks
- At 2 weeks remove splint and begin AROM of elbow and forearm pronosupination
- NWB 0-6 weeks
- At 6 weeks, WBAT and begin PROM

Olecranon Tension Band

Olecranon plate

AROM – Active Range Of Motion
NWB – Non Weight Bearing
ORIF – Open Reduction Internal Fixation
PROM – Passive Range Of Motion
ROM – Range Of Motion

Suggested Readings

Baecher N, Edwards S. Olecranon fractures. J Hand Surg Am 2013;38(3):593–604

Nicolas Lee, MD

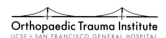

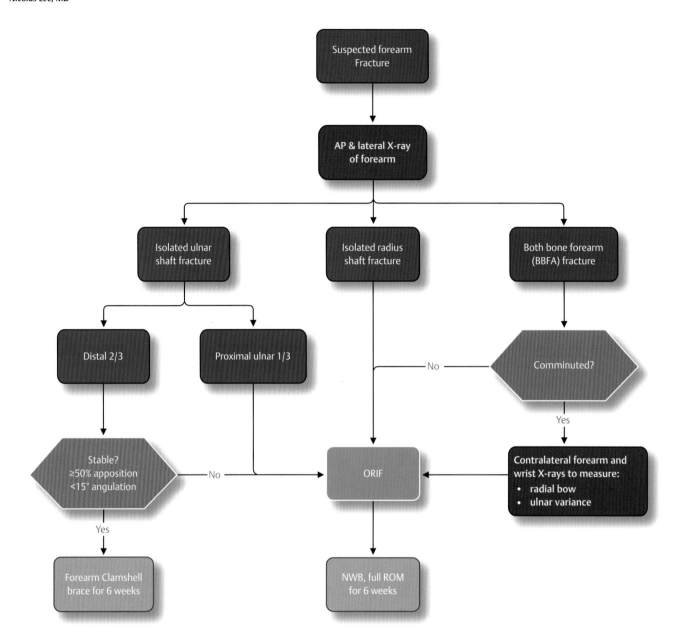

Forearm Clamshell Brace

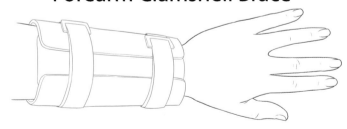

NWB – Non Weight Bearing
ORIF – Open Reduction Internal Fixation
ROM – Range Of Motion

Suggested Readings

Schulte LM, Meals CG, Neviaser RJ. Management of adult diaphyseal both-bone forearm fractures. J Am Acad Orthop Surg 2014;22(7):437–446

Rouleau DM, Sandman E, van Riet R, Galatz LM. Management of fractures of the proximal ulna. J Am Acad Orthop Surg 2013;21(3):149–160

Schemitsch EH, Richards RR. The effect of malunion on functional outcome after plate fixation of fractures of both bones of the forearm in adults. J Bone Joint Surg Am 1992;74(7):1068–1078

Chapter 29: Distal Radius Fractures

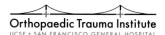

Nicolas Lee, MD

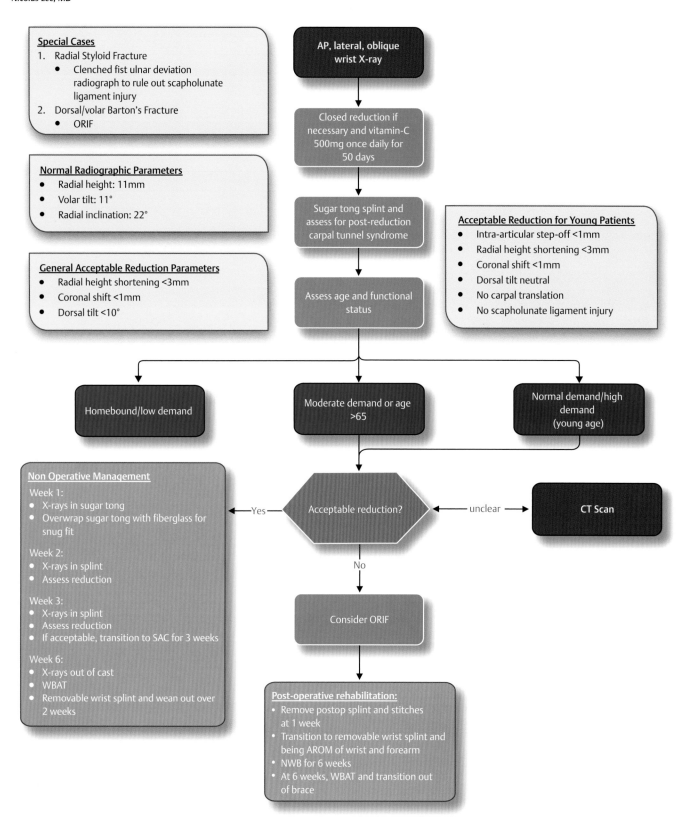

Special Cases
1. Radial Styloid Fracture
   - Clenched fist ulnar deviation radiograph to rule out scapholunate ligament injury
2. Dorsal/volar Barton's Fracture
   - ORIF

Normal Radiographic Parameters
- Radial height: 11mm
- Volar tilt: 11°
- Radial inclination: 22°

General Acceptable Reduction Parameters
- Radial height shortening <3mm
- Coronal shift <1mm
- Dorsal tilt <10°

AP, lateral, oblique wrist X-ray

Closed reduction if necessary and vitamin-C 500mg once daily for 50 days

Sugar tong splint and assess for post-reduction carpal tunnel syndrome

Assess age and functional status

Acceptable Reduction for Young Patients
- Intra-articular step-off <1mm
- Radial height shortening <3mm
- Coronal shift <1mm
- Dorsal tilt neutral
- No carpal translation
- No scapholunate ligament injury

Homebound/low demand

Moderate demand or age >65

Normal demand/high demand (young age)

Non Operative Management

Week 1:
- X-rays in sugar tong
- Overwrap sugar tong with fiberglass for snug fit

Week 2:
- X-rays in splint
- Assess reduction

Week 3:
- X-rays in splint
- Assess reduction
- If acceptable, transition to SAC for 3 weeks

Week 6:
- X-rays out of cast
- WBAT
- Removable wrist splint and wean out over 2 weeks

Acceptable reduction? — Yes / unclear → CT Scan

No

Consider ORIF

Post-operative rehabilitation:
- Remove postop splint and stitches at 1 week
- Transition to removable wrist splint and being AROM of wrist and forearm
- NWB for 6 weeks
- At 6 weeks, WBAT and transition out of brace

Suggested Readings

Murray J, Gross L. Treatment of distal radius fractures. J Am Acad Orthop Surg 2013;21(8):502–505

Koval K, Haidukewych GJ, Service B, Zirgibel BJ. Controversies in the management of distal radius fractures. J Am Acad Orthop Surg 2014;22(9):566–575

Zollinger PE, Tuinebreijer WE, Breederveld RS, Kreis RW. Can vitamin C prevent complex regional pain syndrome in patients with wrist fractures? A randomized, controlled, multicenter dose-response study. J Bone Joint Surg Am 2007;89(7):1424–1431

Chapter 30: Scaphoid Fractures

Nicole Schroeder, MD

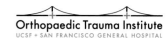

Orthopaedic Trauma Institute
UCSF + SAN FRANCISCO GENERAL HOSPITAL

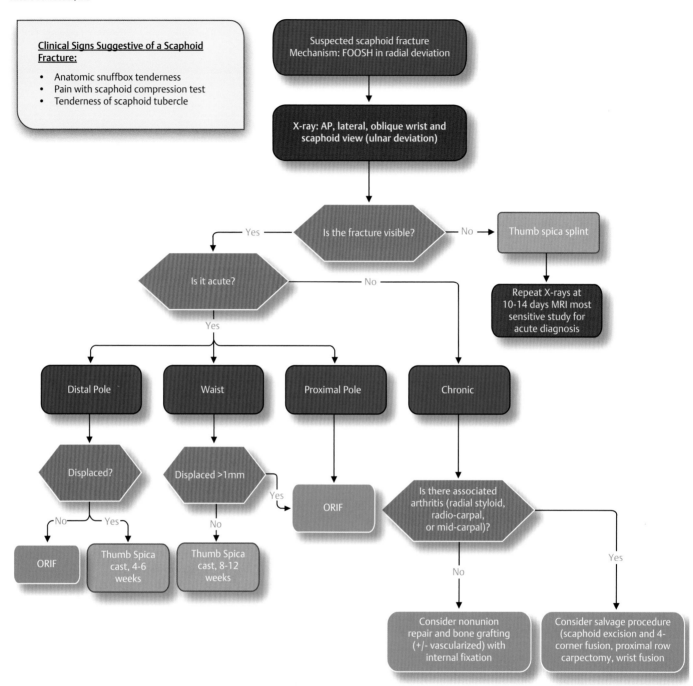

Clinical Signs Suggestive of a Scaphoid Fracture:

- Anatomic snuffbox tenderness
- Pain with scaphoid compression test
- Tenderness of scaphoid tubercle

Suspected scaphoid fracture
Mechanism: FOOSH in radial deviation

X-ray: AP, lateral, oblique wrist and scaphoid view (ulnar deviation)

Is the fracture visible? — No → Thumb spica splint

Thumb spica splint → Repeat X-rays at 10-14 days MRI most sensitive study for acute diagnosis

Yes → Is it acute? — No

Is it acute? Yes →

Distal Pole | Waist | Proximal Pole | Chronic

Distal Pole → Displaced?
Displaced? No → ORIF
Displaced? Yes → Thumb Spica cast, 4-6 weeks

Waist → Displaced >1mm
Displaced >1mm Yes → ORIF
Displaced >1mm No → Thumb Spica cast, 8-12 weeks

Proximal Pole → ORIF

Chronic → Is there associated arthritis (radial styloid, radio-carpal, or mid-carpal)?
No → Consider nonunion repair and bone grafting (+/- vascularized) with internal fixation
Yes → Consider salvage procedure (scaphoid excision and 4-corner fusion, proximal row carpectomy, wrist fusion

FOOSH – Fall on Outstretched Hand
ORIF – Open Reduction Internal Fixation

Chapter 31: Perilunate Dislocation

Nicolas Lee, MD

Orthopaedic Trauma Institute
UCSF + SAN FRANCISCO GENERAL HOSPITAL

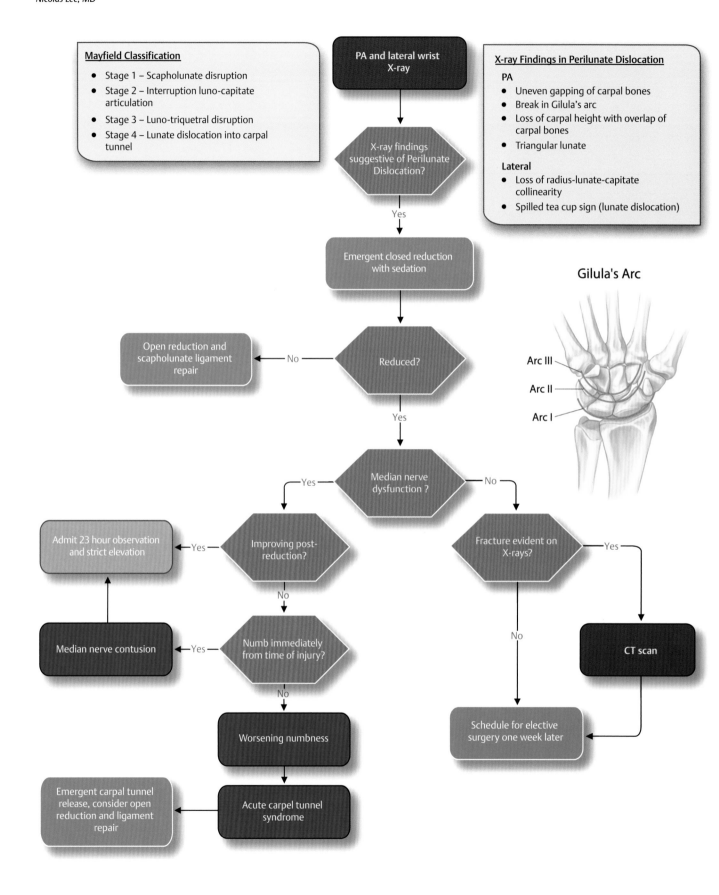

Mayfield Classification

- Stage 1 – Scapholunate disruption
- Stage 2 – Interruption luno-capitate articulation
- Stage 3 – Luno-triquetral disruption
- Stage 4 – Lunate dislocation into carpal tunnel

PA and lateral wrist X-ray

X-ray Findings in Perilunate Dislocation

PA
- Uneven gapping of carpal bones
- Break in Gilula's arc
- Loss of carpal height with overlap of carpal bones
- Triangular lunate

Lateral
- Loss of radius-lunate-capitate collinearity
- Spilled tea cup sign (lunate dislocation)

X-ray findings suggestive of Perilunate Dislocation? — Yes →

Emergent closed reduction with sedation

Reduced? — No → Open reduction and scapholunate ligament repair

Yes →

Gilula's Arc

Arc III
Arc II
Arc I

Median nerve dysfunction ?

Yes → Improving post-reduction?
- Yes → Admit 23 hour observation and strict elevation
- No → Numb immediately from time of injury?
  - Yes → Median nerve contusion → Admit 23 hour observation and strict elevation
  - No → Worsening numbness → Acute carpel tunnel syndrome → Emergent carpal tunnel release, consider open reduction and ligament repair

No → Fracture evident on X-rays?
- Yes → CT scan → Schedule for elective surgery one week later
- No → Schedule for elective surgery one week later

Suggested Readings

Stanbury SJ, Elfar JC. Perilunate dislocation and perilunate fracture-dislocation. J Am Acad Orthop Surg 2011;19(9):554–562

Chapter 32: Extensor Tendon Lacerations

Nicole Schroeder, MD

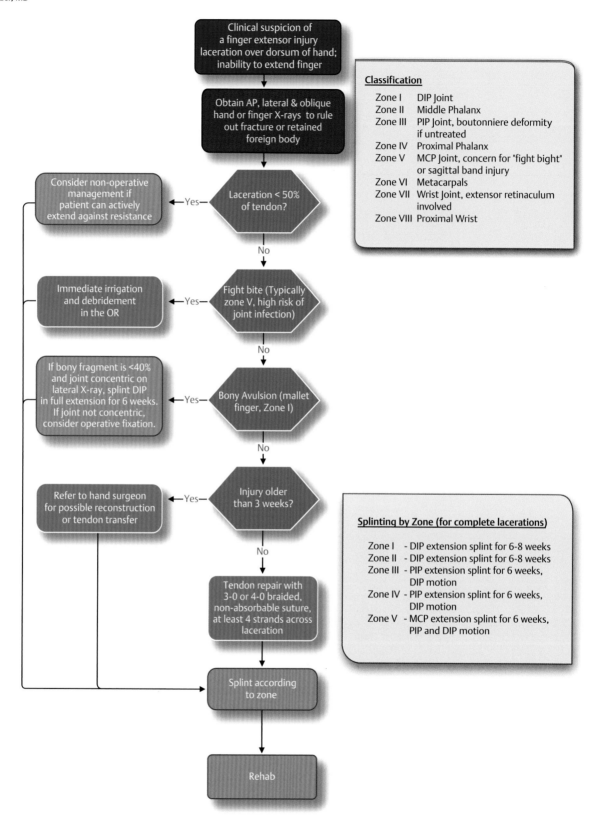

Clinical suspicion of a finger extensor injury laceration over dorsum of hand; inability to extend finger

Obtain AP, lateral & oblique hand or finger X-rays to rule out fracture or retained foreign body

Laceration < 50% of tendon? —Yes→ **Consider non-operative management if patient can actively extend against resistance**

No

Fight bite (Typically zone V, high risk of joint infection) —Yes→ **Immediate irrigation and debridement in the OR**

No

Bony Avulsion (mallet finger, Zone I) —Yes→ **If bony fragment is <40% and joint concentric on lateral X-ray, splint DIP in full extension for 6 weeks. If joint not concentric, consider operative fixation.**

No

Injury older than 3 weeks? —Yes→ **Refer to hand surgeon for possible reconstruction or tendon transfer**

No

Tendon repair with 3-0 or 4-0 braided, non-absorbable suture, at least 4 strands across laceration

Splint according to zone

Rehab

Classification

Zone I	DIP Joint
Zone II	Middle Phalanx
Zone III	PIP Joint, boutonniere deformity if untreated
Zone IV	Proximal Phalanx
Zone V	MCP Joint, concern for "fight bight" or sagittal band injury
Zone VI	Metacarpals
Zone VII	Wrist Joint, extensor retinaculum involved
Zone VIII	Proximal Wrist

Splinting by Zone (for complete lacerations)

Zone I	- DIP extension splint for 6-8 weeks
Zone II	- DIP extension splint for 6-8 weeks
Zone III	- PIP extension splint for 6 weeks, DIP motion
Zone IV	- PIP extension splint for 6 weeks, DIP motion
Zone V	- MCP extension splint for 6 weeks, PIP and DIP motion

DIP – Distal interphalangeal (joint)
PIP – Proximal interphalangeal (joint)
MCP – Metacarpophalangeal (joint)

Suggested Readings

Matzon JL, Bozentka DJ. Extensor tendon injuries. The Journal of hand surgery. 2010 May 31;35(5):854-61.

Amirtharajah M, Lattanza L. Open extensor tendon injuries. The Journal of hand surgery. 2015 Feb 28a;40(2):391-7.

Chapter 33: Flexor Tendon Injuries

Nicole Schroeder, MD

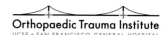
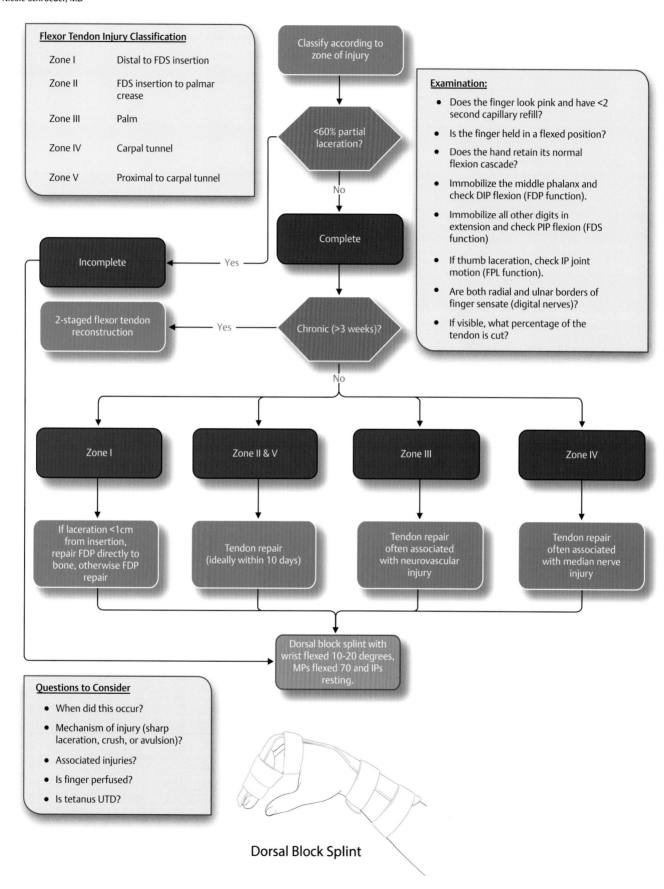

Flexor Tendon Injury Classification

Zone I	Distal to FDS insertion
Zone II	FDS insertion to palmar crease
Zone III	Palm
Zone IV	Carpal tunnel
Zone V	Proximal to carpal tunnel

Classify according to zone of injury

<60% partial laceration?

Complete

— No

Incomplete ←— Yes

2-staged flexor tendon reconstruction ←— Yes — Chronic (>3 weeks)?

— No

Examination:

- Does the finger look pink and have <2 second capillary refill?
- Is the finger held in a flexed position?
- Does the hand retain its normal flexion cascade?
- Immobilize the middle phalanx and check DIP flexion (FDP function).
- Immobilize all other digits in extension and check PIP flexion (FDS function)
- If thumb laceration, check IP joint motion (FPL function).
- Are both radial and ulnar borders of finger sensate (digital nerves)?
- If visible, what percentage of the tendon is cut?

Zone I

If laceration <1cm from insertion, repair FDP directly to bone, otherwise FDP repair

Zone II & V

Tendon repair (ideally within 10 days)

Zone III

Tendon repair often associated with neurovascular injury

Zone IV

Tendon repair often associated with median nerve injury

Dorsal block splint with wrist flexed 10-20 degrees, MPs flexed 70 and IPs resting.

Questions to Consider

- When did this occur?
- Mechanism of injury (sharp laceration, crush, or avulsion)?
- Associated injuries?
- Is finger perfused?
- Is tetanus UTD?

Dorsal Block Splint

Suggested Readings

Boyer MI, Strickland JW, Engles D, Sachar K, Leversedge FJ. Flexor tendon repair and rehabilitation: state of the art in 2002. Instr Course Lect

Chapter 34: Finger Replantation

Nicole Schroeder, MD

Indications for Replantation
- Multiple digits
- Thumb
- Through the palm, wrist, or proximal
- Amputated digit in child

Relative Indications
- Digit distal to Zone II
- Ring avulsion
- Through or above elbow

Contraindications
- Severe vascular disorder
- Mangled limb
- Segmental amputation

Relative contraindications
- Medically unstable patient
- Severe psychiatric illness
- Prolonged warm ischemia time
- Tissue contamination

Questions to Consider for Replantation
- How long ago did this happen?
- What was the exact mechanism of injury (crush, avulsion, sharp transection, etc.)?
- Medical comorbidities
- Is your hospital equipped for replantation surgery? If not consider transfer to select hospitals.

Traumatic finger amputation

↓

Wrap amputated part in moist gauze, place in bag, and place bag in ice. Apply direct pressure and dressing (not tourniquet) to wound to stop bleeding.
Provide IV antibiotics, check tetanus status.

↓

X-ray: AP/lateral/oblique of hand and amputated digit

↓

Does my hospital have replantation service? —No→

Transfer to replantation facility:
- Include any salvageable tissue
- Tissue wrapped in moist gauze
- Place in sealed bag in ice

Yes ↓

Is replantation indicated?

Yes ↓

Are there any contraindications?

No ↓

Warm ischemia <12 hours?
Cold ischemia <24 hours?

Yes ↓

Perform replantation

↓

Keep patient in warm room
Avoid: caffeine, chocolate, nicotine

↓

Monitor skin temperature and pulse oximetry

Suggested Readings

Wolfe VM, Wang AA. Replantation of the upper extremity: current concepts. J Am Acad Orthop Surg 2015;23(6):373–381

Chapter 35: Finger Fractures

Nicole Schroeder, MD

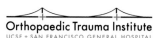
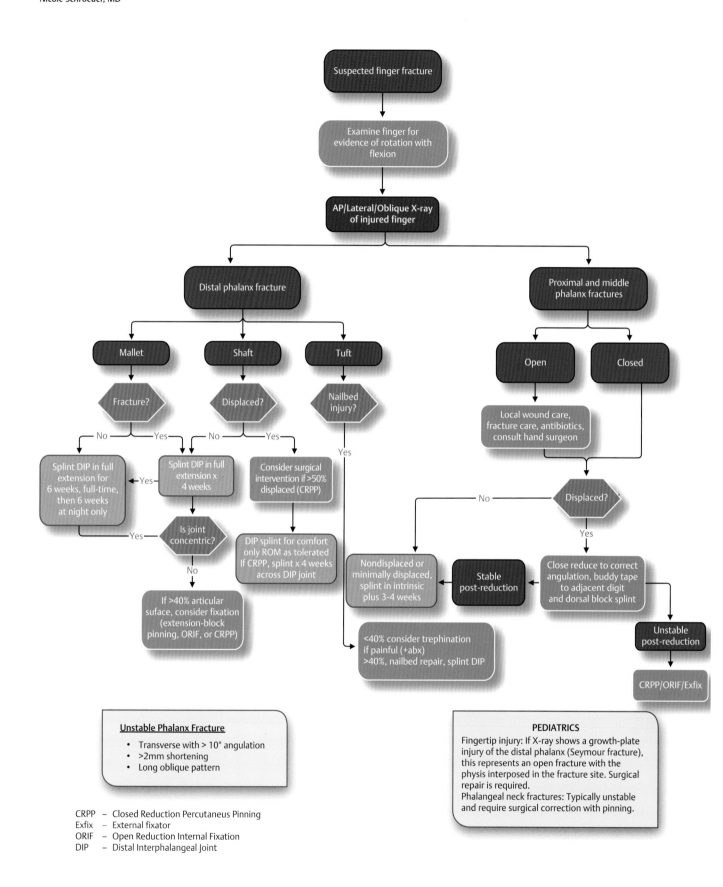

Suspected finger fracture

Examine finger for evidence of rotation with flexion

AP/Lateral/Oblique X-ray of injured finger

Distal phalanx fracture

Proximal and middle phalanx fractures

Mallet — Fracture?
- No
- Yes

Shaft — Displaced?
- No
- Yes

Tuft — Nailbed injury?
- Yes

Open

Closed

Splint DIP in full extension for 6 weeks, full-time, then 6 weeks at night only

Splint DIP in full extension x 4 weeks — Yes

Consider surgical intervention if >50% displaced (CRPP)

Local wound care, fracture care, antibiotics, consult hand surgeon

Is joint concentric? — Yes / No

DIP splint for comfort only ROM as tolerated If CRPP, splint x 4 weeks across DIP joint

Displaced? — No / Yes

If >40% articular suface, consider fixation (extension-block pinning, ORIF, or CRPP)

Nondisplaced or minimally displaced, splint in intrinsic plus 3-4 weeks

Stable post-reduction

Close reduce to correct angulation, buddy tape to adjacent digit and dorsal block splint

<40% consider trephination if painful (+abx) >40%, nailbed repair, splint DIP

Unstable post-reduction

CRPP/ORIF/Exfix

Unstable Phalanx Fracture

- Transverse with > 10° angulation
- >2mm shortening
- Long oblique pattern

PEDIATRICS

Fingertip injury: If X-ray shows a growth-plate injury of the distal phalanx (Seymour fracture), this represents an open fracture with the physis interposed in the fracture site. Surgical repair is required.

Phalangeal neck fractures: Typically unstable and require surgical correction with pinning.

CRPP – Closed Reduction Percutaneus Pinning
Exfix – External fixator
ORIF – Open Reduction Internal Fixation
DIP – Distal Interphalangeal Joint

Suggested Readings

Abzug JM, Dua K, Bauer AS, Cornwall R, Wyrick TO. Pediatric Phalanx Fractures. J Am Acad Orthop Surg 2016;24(11):e174–e183

Meals C, Meals R. Hand fractures: a review of current treatment strategies. J Hand Surg Am 2013;38(5):1021–1031, quiz 1031

Chapter 36: Metacarpal Fractures

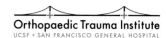

Nicole Schroeder, MD

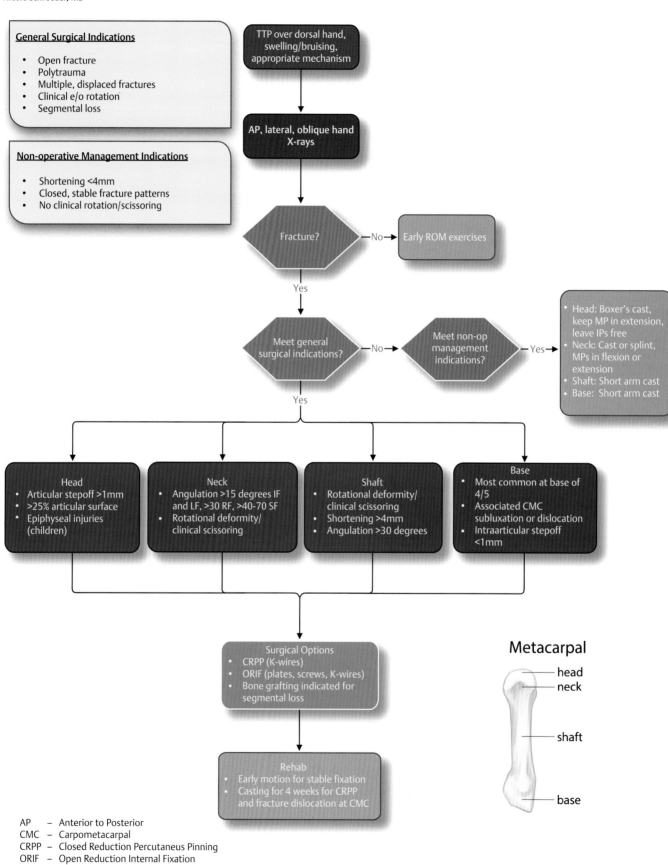

General Surgical Indications

- Open fracture
- Polytrauma
- Multiple, displaced fractures
- Clinical e/o rotation
- Segmental loss

Non-operative Management Indications

- Shortening <4mm
- Closed, stable fracture patterns
- No clinical rotation/scissoring

TTP over dorsal hand, swelling/bruising, appropriate mechanism

AP, lateral, oblique hand X-rays

Fracture? — No → Early ROM exercises

Yes

Meet general surgical indications? — No → Meet non-op management indications? — Yes →
- Head: Boxer's cast, keep MP in extension, leave IPs free
- Neck: Cast or splint, MPs in flexion or extension
- Shaft: Short arm cast
- Base: Short arm cast

Yes

Head
- Articular stepoff >1mm
- >25% articular surface
- Epiphyseal injuries (children)

Neck
- Angulation >15 degrees IF and LF, >30 RF, >40-70 SF
- Rotational deformity/ clinical scissoring

Shaft
- Rotational deformity/ clinical scissoring
- Shortening >4mm
- Angulation >30 degrees

Base
- Most common at base of 4/5
- Associated CMC subluxation or dislocation
- Intraarticular stepoff <1mm

Surgical Options
- CRPP (K-wires)
- ORIF (plates, screws, K-wires)
- Bone grafting indicated for segmental loss

Rehab
- Early motion for stable fixation
- Casting for 4 weeks for CRPP and fracture dislocation at CMC

Metacarpal
- head
- neck
- shaft
- base

AP   –   Anterior to Posterior
CMC   –   Carpometacarpal
CRPP   –   Closed Reduction Percutaneus Pinning
ORIF   –   Open Reduction Internal Fixation
TTP   –   Tender To Palpation

Chapter 37: Metacarpophalangeal (MCP) Dislocations

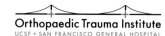

Nicole Schroeder, MD

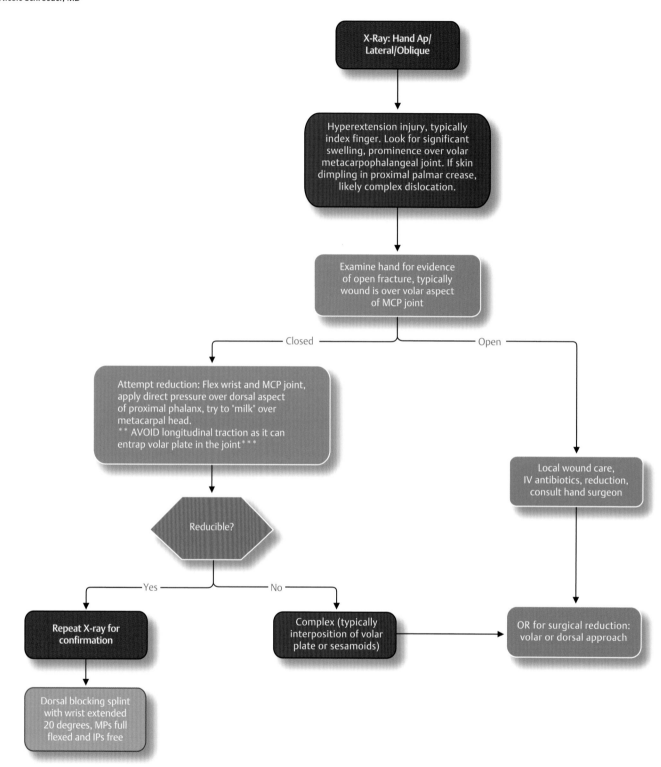

MP – Metacarpophalangel joint
IP – Interphalangeal joint

Suggested Readings

Dinh P, Franklin A, Hutchinson B, Schnall SB, Fassola I. Metacarpophalangeal joint dislocation. J Am Acad Orthop Surg 2009;17(5):318–324

Chapter 38: Phalanx Dislocations

Orthopaedic Trauma Institute
UCSF + SAN FRANCISCO GENERAL HOSPITAL

Nicole Schroeder, MD

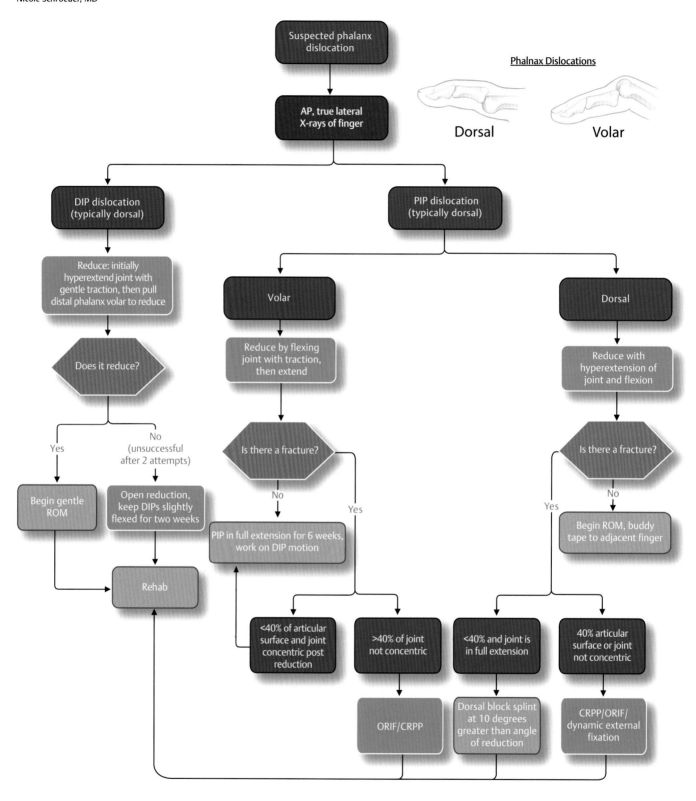

Phalnax Dislocations

Dorsal   Volar

Suspected phalanx dislocation

AP, true lateral X-rays of finger

DIP dislocation (typically dorsal)

PIP dislocation (typically dorsal)

Reduce: initially hyperextend joint with gentle traction, then pull distal phalanx volar to reduce

Volar

Dorsal

Does it reduce?

Reduce by flexing joint with traction, then extend

Reduce with hyperextension of joint and flexion

Yes

No (unsuccessful after 2 attempts)

Is there a fracture?

Is there a fracture?

Begin gentle ROM

Open reduction, keep DIPs slightly flexed for two weeks

No

Yes

No

Yes

PIP in full extension for 6 weeks, work on DIP motion

Begin ROM, buddy tape to adjacent finger

Rehab

<40% of articular surface and joint concentric post reduction

>40% of joint not concentric

<40% and joint is in full extension

40% articular surface or joint not concentric

ORIF/CRPP

Dorsal block splint at 10 degrees greater than angle of reduction

CRPP/ORIF/ dynamic external fixation

DIP – Distal interphalangeal (joint)
PIP – Proximal interphalangeal (joint)

Suggested Readings

Borchers JR, Best TM. Common finger fractures and dislocations. American family physician. 2012 Apr 15;85(8).

Chapter 39: Femoral Shaft Fractures

R. Trigg McClellan, MD

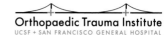

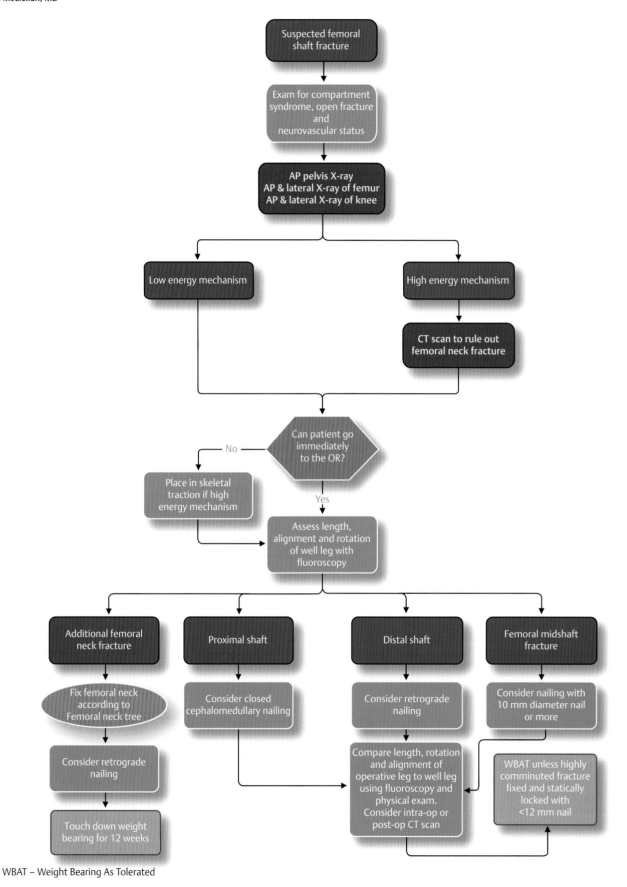

WBAT – Weight Bearing As Tolerated

Suggested Readings

Tornetta P III, Kain MS, Creevy WR. Diagnosis of femoral neck fractures in patients with a femoral shaft fracture. Improvement with a standard protocol. J Bone Joint Surg Am 2007;89(1):39–43

Brumback RJ, Toal TR Jr, Murphy-Zane MS, Novak VP, Belkoff SM. Immediate weight-bearing after treatment of a comminuted fracture of the femoral shaft with a statically locked intramedullary nail. J Bone Joint Surg Am 1999;81(11):1538–1544

Krettek C, Miclau T, Grün O, Schandelmaier P, Tscherne H. Intraoperative control of axes, rotation and length in femoral and tibial fractures. Technical note. Injury 1998;29(Suppl 3):C29–C39

Chapter 40: Distal Femur Fractures

Paul Toogood, MD

Orthopaedic Trauma Institute
UCSF + SAN FRANCISCO GENERAL HOSPITAL

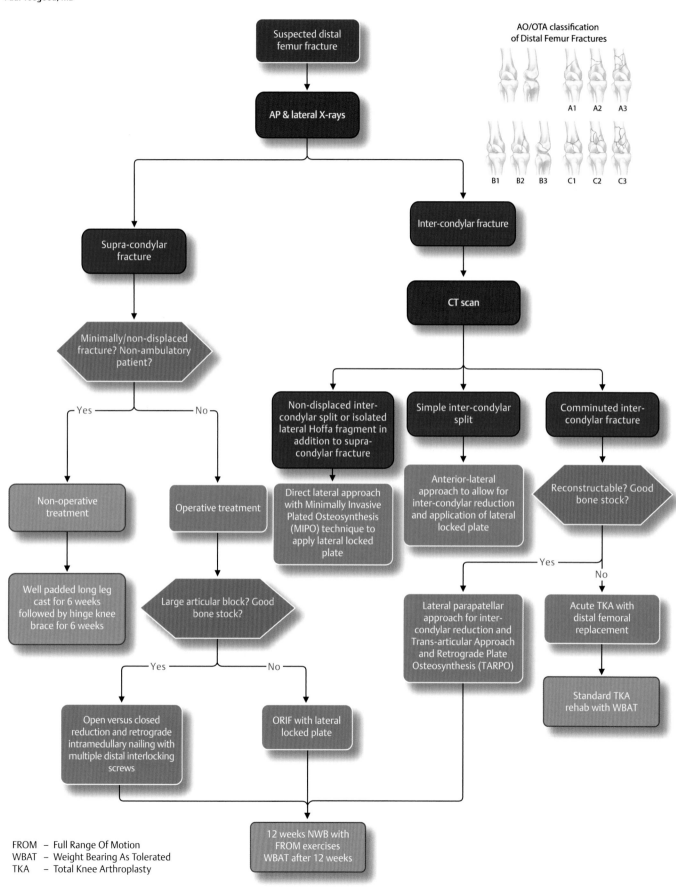

AO/OTA classification of Distal Femur Fractures

A1 A2 A3

B1 B2 B3 C1 C2 C3

Suspected distal femur fracture

AP & lateral X-rays

Supra-condylar fracture

Inter-condylar fracture

CT scan

Minimally/non-displaced fracture? Non-ambulatory patient?

Non-displaced inter-condylar split or isolated lateral Hoffa fragment in addition to supra-condylar fracture

Simple inter-condylar split

Comminuted inter-condylar fracture

Yes → Non-operative treatment

No → Operative treatment

Direct lateral approach with Minimally Invasive Plated Osteosynthesis (MIPO) technique to apply lateral locked plate

Anterior-lateral approach to allow for inter-condylar reduction and application of lateral locked plate

Reconstructable? Good bone stock?

Well padded long leg cast for 6 weeks followed by hinge knee brace for 6 weeks

Large articular block? Good bone stock?

Lateral parapatellar approach for inter-condylar reduction and Trans-articular Approach and Retrograde Plate Osteosynthesis (TARPO)

Yes →

No → Acute TKA with distal femoral replacement

Yes → Open versus closed reduction and retrograde intramedullary nailing with multiple distal interlocking screws

No → ORIF with lateral locked plate

Standard TKA rehab with WBAT

12 weeks NWB with FROM exercises WBAT after 12 weeks

FROM – Full Range Of Motion
WBAT – Weight Bearing As Tolerated
TKA – Total Knee Arthroplasty

Suggested Readings

Nork SE, Segina DN, Aflatoon K, et al. The association between supracondylar-intercondylar distal femoral fractures and coronal plane fractures. J Bone Joint Surg Am 2005;87(3):564–569

Rodriguez EK, Zurakowski D, Herder L, et al. Mechanical Construct Characteristics Predisposing To Non-Union After Locked Lateral Plating Of Distal Femur Fractures. J Orthop Trauma 2016; 30(8):403–8

Krettek C, Schandelmaier P, Miclau T, Bertram R, Holmes W, Tscherne H. Transarticular joint reconstruction and indirect plate osteosynthesis for complex distal supracondylar femoral fractures. Injury 1997;28(Suppl 1):A31–A41 Review

Krettek C, Müller M, Miclau T. Evolution of minimally invasive plate osteosynthesis (MIPO) in the femur. Injury 2001;32(Suppl 3):SC14–SC23 Review

Starr AJ, Jones AL, Reinert CM. The "swashbuckler": a modified anterior approach for fractures of the distal femur. J Orthop Trauma 1999;13(2):138–140

Freedman EL, Hak DJ, Johnson EE, Eckardt JJ. Total knee replacement including a modular distal femoral component in elderly patients with acute fracture or nonunion. J Orthop Trauma 1995;9(3):231–237

Chapter 41: Traumatic Knee Dislocation

Utku Kandemir, MD

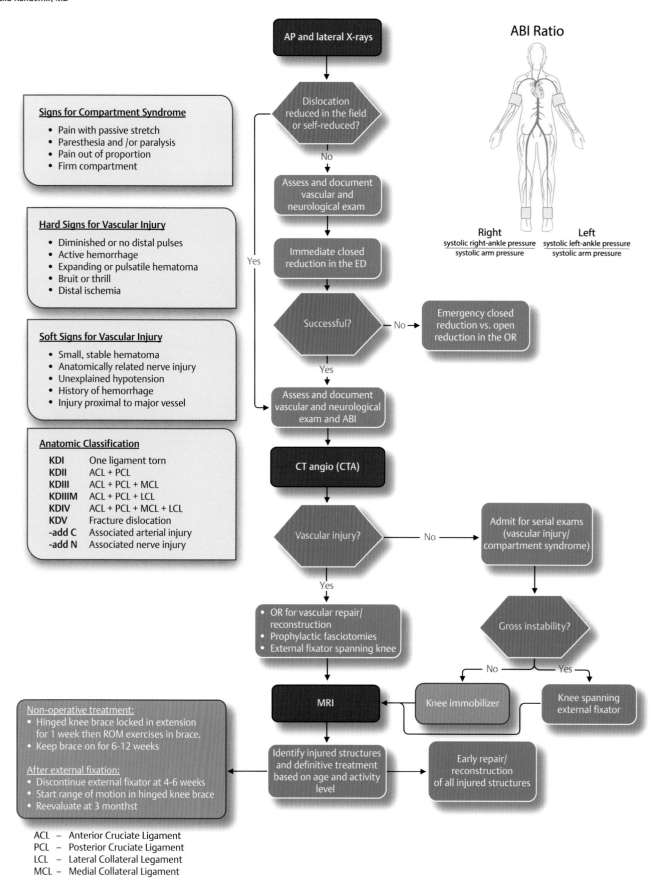

ABI Ratio

Right
$$\frac{\text{systolic right-ankle pressure}}{\text{systolic arm pressure}}$$

Left
$$\frac{\text{systolic left-ankle pressure}}{\text{systolic arm pressure}}$$

AP and lateral X-rays

Dislocation reduced in the field or self-reduced? — Yes / No

Assess and document vascular and neurological exam

Immediate closed reduction in the ED

Successful? — No → Emergency closed reduction vs. open reduction in the OR

Yes → Assess and document vascular and neurological exam and ABI

CT angio (CTA)

Vascular injury? — No → Admit for serial exams (vascular injury/compartment syndrome)

Yes →
- OR for vascular repair/reconstruction
- Prophylactic fasciotomies
- External fixator spanning knee

Gross instability? — No → Knee immobilizer / Yes → Knee spanning external fixator

MRI

Identify injured structures and definitive treatment based on age and activity level → Early repair/reconstruction of all injured structures

Signs for Compartment Syndrome
- Pain with passive stretch
- Paresthesia and /or paralysis
- Pain out of proportion
- Firm compartment

Hard Signs for Vascular Injury
- Diminished or no distal pulses
- Active hemorrhage
- Expanding or pulsatile hematoma
- Bruit or thrill
- Distal ischemia

Soft Signs for Vascular Injury
- Small, stable hematoma
- Anatomically related nerve injury
- Unexplained hypotension
- History of hemorrhage
- Injury proximal to major vessel

Anatomic Classification
KDI	One ligament torn
KDII	ACL + PCL
KDIII	ACL + PCL + MCL
KDIIIM	ACL + PCL + LCL
KDIV	ACL + PCL + MCL + LCL
KDV	Fracture dislocation
-add C	Associated arterial injury
-add N	Associated nerve injury

Non-operative treatment:
- Hinged knee brace locked in extension for 1 week then ROM exercises in brace.
- Keep brace on for 6-12 weeks

After external fixation:
- Discontinue external fixator at 4-6 weeks
- Start range of motion in hinged knee brace
- Reevaluate at 3 monthst

ACL – Anterior Cruciate Ligament
PCL – Posterior Cruciate Ligament
LCL – Lateral Collateral Legament
MCL – Medial Collateral Ligament

Suggested Readings

Schenck RC Jr. The dislocated knee. Instr Course Lect 1994;43:127–136

Chapter 42: Patella Fractures

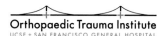
Orthopaedic Trauma Institute
UCSF + SAN FRANCISCO GENERAL HOSPITAL

Meir T. Marmor, MD

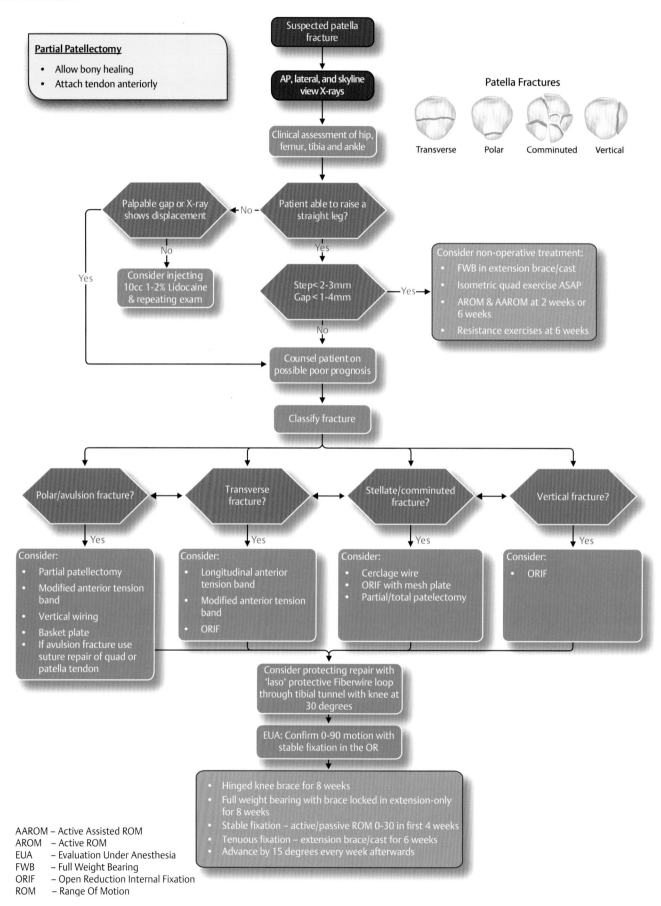

Partial Patellectomy
- Allow bony healing
- Attach tendon anteriorly

Suspected patella fracture

AP, lateral, and skyline view X-rays

Clinical assessment of hip, femur, tibia and ankle

Patella Fractures

Transverse   Polar   Comminuted   Vertical

Patient able to raise a straight leg?

Palpable gap or X-ray shows displacement — No

No → Consider injecting 10cc 1-2% Lidocaine & repeating exam

Yes

Step < 2-3mm Gap < 1-4mm — Yes →

Consider non-operative treatment:
- FWB in extension brace/cast
- Isometric quad exercise ASAP
- AROM & AAROM at 2 weeks or 6 weeks
- Resistance exercises at 6 weeks

No

Counsel patient on possible poor prognosis

Classify fracture

Polar/avulsion fracture? — Yes

Consider:
- Partial patellectomy
- Modified anterior tension band
- Vertical wiring
- Basket plate
- If avulsion fracture use suture repair of quad or patella tendon

Transverse fracture? — Yes

Consider:
- Longitudinal anterior tension band
- Modified anterior tension band
- ORIF

Stellate/comminuted fracture? — Yes

Consider:
- Cerclage wire
- ORIF with mesh plate
- Partial/total patelectomy

Vertical fracture? — Yes

Consider:
- ORIF

Consider protecting repair with 'laso' protective Fiberwire loop through tibial tunnel with knee at 30 degrees

EUA: Confirm 0-90 motion with stable fixation in the OR

- Hinged knee brace for 8 weeks
- Full weight bearing with brace locked in extension-only for 8 weeks
- Stable fixation – active/passive ROM 0-30 in first 4 weeks
- Tenuous fixation – extension brace/cast for 6 weeks
- Advance by 15 degrees every week afterwards

AAROM – Active Assisted ROM
AROM – Active ROM
EUA   – Evaluation Under Anesthesia
FWB   – Full Weight Bearing
ORIF   – Open Reduction Internal Fixation
ROM   – Range Of Motion

Suggested Readings

Marder RA, Swanson TV, Sharkey NA, Duwelius PJ. Effects of partial patellectomy and reattachment of the patellar tendon on patellofemoral contact areas and pressures. J Bone Joint Surg Am 1993;75(1):35–45

LeBrun CT, Langford JR, Sagi HC. Functional outcomes after operatively treated patella fractures. J Orthop Trauma 2012;26(7):422–426

Berg EE. Open reduction internal fixation of displaced transverse patella fractures with figure-eight wiring through parallel cannulated compression screws. J Orthop Trauma 1997;11(8):573–576

Carpenter JE, Kasman RA, Patel N, Lee ML, Goldstein SA. Biomechanical evaluation of current patella fracture fixation techniques. J Orthop Trauma 1997;11(5):351–356

West JL, Keene JS, Kaplan LD. Early motion after quadriceps and patellar tendon repairs: outcomes with single-suture augmentation. Am J Sports Med 2008;36(2):316–323

Boström A. Fracture of the patella. A study of 422 patellar fractures. Acta Orthop Scand Suppl 1972;143:1–80

Kim YM, Yang JY, Kim KC, et al. Separate Vertical Wirings for the Extra-articular Fractures of the Distal Pole of the Patella. Knee Surg Relat Res 2011;23(4):220–226

Kastelec M, Veselko M. Inferior patellar pole avulsion fractures: osteosynthesis compared with pole resection. J Bone Joint Surg Am 2004;86-A(4):696–701

Melvin JS, Mehta S. Patellar fractures in adults. J Am Acad Orthop Surg 2011;19(4):198–207

West JL, Keene JS, Kaplan LD. Early motion after quadriceps and patellar tendon repairs: outcomes with single-suture augmentation. Am J Sports Med 2008;36(2):316–323

Orthopaedic Trauma Institute
UCSF • SAN FRANCISCO GENERAL HOSPITAL

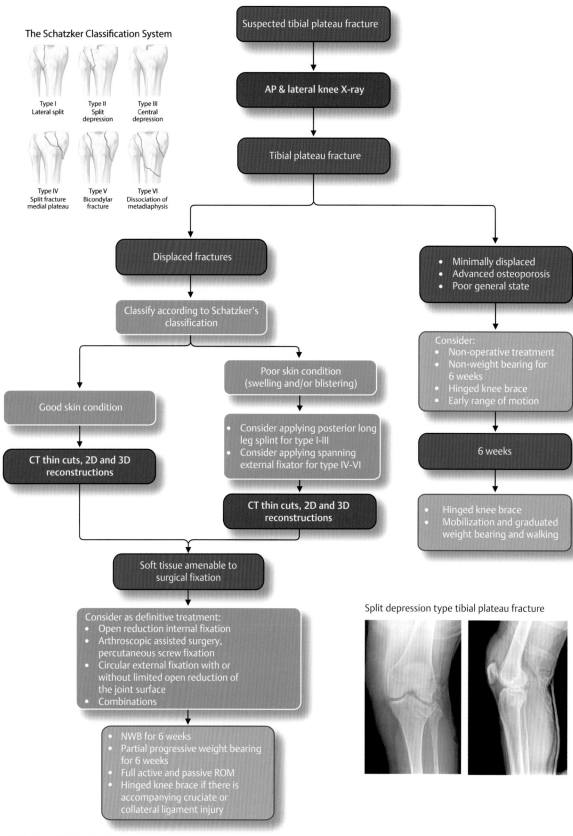

The Schatzker Classification System

Type I
Lateral split

Type II
Split depression

Type III
Central depression

Type IV
Split fracture medial plateau

Type V
Bicondylar fracture

Type VI
Dissociation of metadiaphysis

Suspected tibial plateau fracture

AP & lateral knee X-ray

Tibial plateau fracture

Displaced fractures

Classify according to Schatzker's classification

Good skin condition

CT thin cuts, 2D and 3D reconstructions

Poor skin condition (swelling and/or blistering)

- Consider applying posterior long leg splint for type I-III
- Consider applying spanning external fixator for type IV-VI

CT thin cuts, 2D and 3D reconstructions

Soft tissue amenable to surgical fixation

Consider as definitive treatment:
- Open reduction internal fixation
- Arthroscopic assisted surgery, percutaneous screw fixation
- Circular external fixation with or without limited open reduction of the joint surface
- Combinations

- NWB for 6 weeks
- Partial progressive weight bearing for 6 weeks
- Full active and passive ROM
- Hinged knee brace if there is accompanying cruciate or collateral ligament injury

- Minimally displaced
- Advanced osteoporosis
- Poor general state

Consider:
- Non-operative treatment
- Non-weight bearing for 6 weeks
- Hinged knee brace
- Early range of motion

6 weeks

- Hinged knee brace
- Mobilization and graduated weight bearing and walking

Split depression type tibial plateau fracture

NWB – Non Weight Bearing
ROM – Range Of Motion

Suggested Readings

Schatzker J, McBroom R, Bruce D. The tibial plateau fracture. The Toronto experience 1968--1975. Clin Orthop Relat Res 1979; (138):94–104

Chapter 44: Tibial Shaft Fractures

R. Trigg McClellan, MD

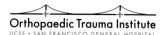

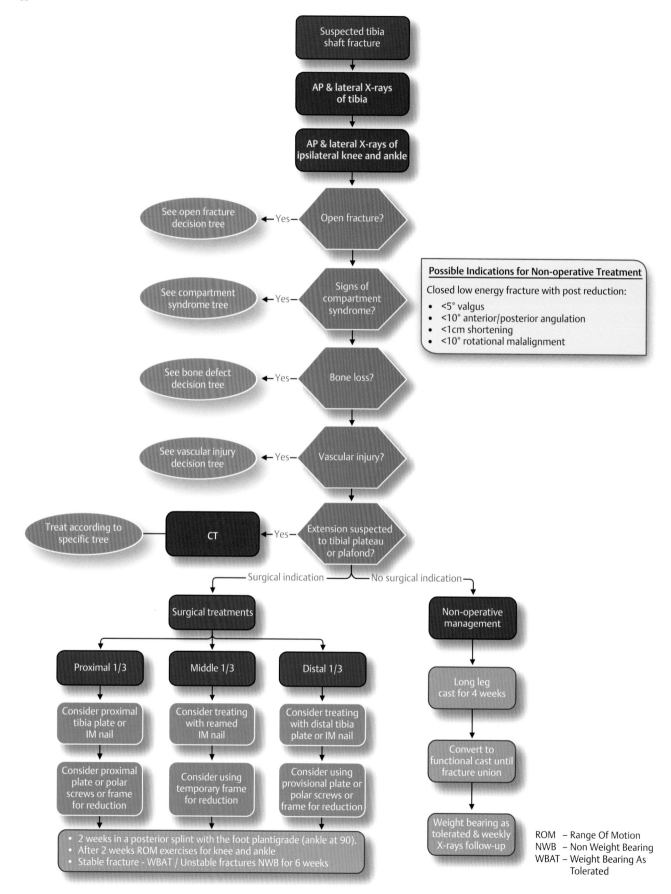

Suspected tibia shaft fracture

AP & lateral X-rays of tibia

AP & lateral X-rays of ipsilateral knee and ankle

Open fracture? —Yes→ See open fracture decision tree

Signs of compartment syndrome? —Yes→ See compartment syndrome tree

Possible Indications for Non-operative Treatment

Closed low energy fracture with post reduction:
- <5° valgus
- <10° anterior/posterior angulation
- <1cm shortening
- <10° rotational malalignment

Bone loss? —Yes→ See bone defect decision tree

Vascular injury? —Yes→ See vascular injury decision tree

Extension suspected to tibial plateau or plafond? —Yes→ CT — Treat according to specific tree

Surgical indication / No surgical indication

Surgical treatments

Non-operative management

Proximal 1/3
Consider proximal tibia plate or IM nail
Consider proximal plate or polar screws or frame for reduction

Middle 1/3
Consider treating with reamed IM nail
Consider using temporary frame for reduction

Distal 1/3
Consider treating with distal tibia plate or IM nail
Consider using provisional plate or polar screws or frame for reduction

- 2 weeks in a posterior splint with the foot plantigrade (ankle at 90).
- After 2 weeks ROM exercises for knee and ankle
- Stable fracture - WBAT / Unstable fractures NWB for 6 weeks

Long leg cast for 4 weeks

Convert to functional cast until fracture union

Weight bearing as tolerated & weekly X-rays follow-up

ROM – Range Of Motion
NWB – Non Weight Bearing
WBAT – Weight Bearing As Tolerated

Suggested Readings

Sarmiento A, Gersten LM, Sobol PA, Shankwiler JA, Vangsness CT. Tibial shaft fractures treated with functional braces. Experience with 780 fractures. J Bone Joint Surg Br 1989;71(4):602–609

R. Trigg McClellan, MD

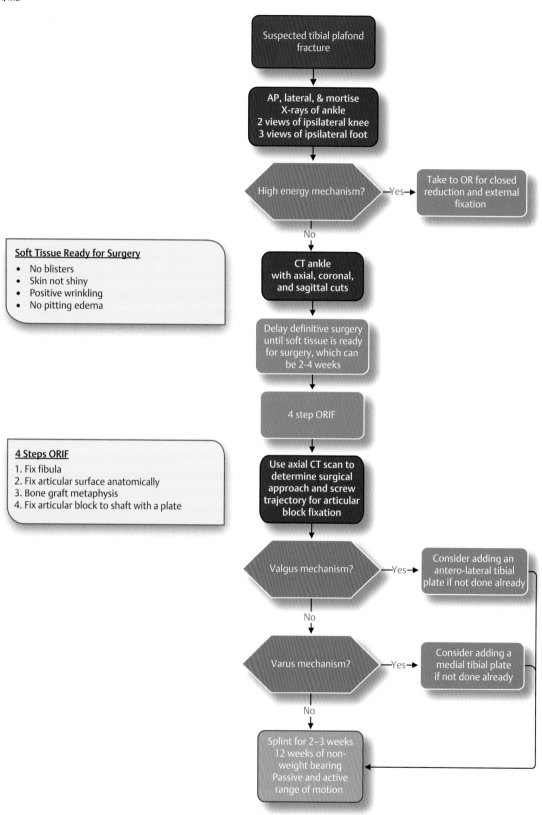

Soft Tissue Ready for Surgery

- No blisters
- Skin not shiny
- Positive wrinkling
- No pitting edema

4 Steps ORIF

1. Fix fibula
2. Fix articular surface anatomically
3. Bone graft metaphysis
4. Fix articular block to shaft with a plate

Suspected tibial plafond fracture

AP, lateral, & mortise X-rays of ankle
2 views of ipsilateral knee
3 views of ipsilateral foot

High energy mechanism? —Yes→ Take to OR for closed reduction and external fixation

No

CT ankle with axial, coronal, and sagittal cuts

Delay definitive surgery until soft tissue is ready for surgery, which can be 2-4 weeks

4 step ORIF

Use axial CT scan to determine surgical approach and screw trajectory for articular block fixation

Valgus mechanism? —Yes→ Consider adding an antero-lateral tibial plate if not done already

No

Varus mechanism? —Yes→ Consider adding a medial tibial plate if not done already

No

Splint for 2–3 weeks
12 weeks of non-weight bearing
Passive and active range of motion

Suggested Readings

Sirkin M, Sanders R, DiPasquale T, Herscovici D Jr. A staged protocol for soft tissue management in the treatment of complex pilon fractures. J Orthop Trauma 1999;13(2):78–84

Rüedi TP, Allgöwer M. The operative treatment of intra-articular fractures of the lower end of the tibia. Clin Orthop Relat Res 1979; (138):105–110

Chapter 46: Ankle Fractures

Meir T. Marmor, MD

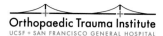

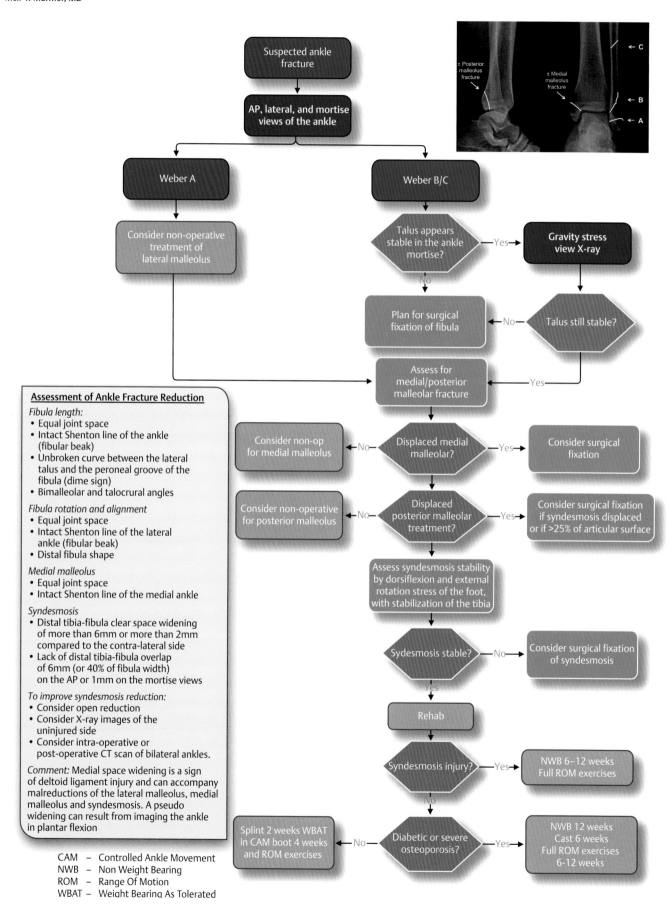

Assessment of Ankle Fracture Reduction

Fibula length:
- Equal joint space
- Intact Shenton line of the ankle (fibular beak)
- Unbroken curve between the lateral talus and the peroneal groove of the fibula (dime sign)
- Bimalleolar and talocrural angles

Fibula rotation and alignment
- Equal joint space
- Intact Shenton line of the lateral ankle (fibular beak)
- Distal fibula shape

Medial malleolus
- Equal joint space
- Intact Shenton line of the medial ankle

Syndesmosis
- Distal tibia-fibula clear space widening of more than 6mm or more than 2mm compared to the contra-lateral side
- Lack of distal tibia-fibula overlap of 6mm (or 40% of fibula width) on the AP or 1mm on the mortise views

To improve syndesmosis reduction:
- Consider open reduction
- Consider X-ray images of the uninjured side
- Consider intra-operative or post-operative CT scan of bilateral ankles.

Comment: Medial space widening is a sign of deltoid ligament injury and can accompany malreductions of the lateral malleolus, medial malleolus and syndesmosis. A pseudo widening can result from imaging the ankle in plantar flexion

CAM – Controlled Ankle Movement
NWB – Non Weight Bearing
ROM – Range Of Motion
WBAT – Weight Bearing As Tolerated

Suggested Readings

Gill JB, Risko T, Raducan V, Grimes JS, Schutt RC Jr. Comparison of manual and gravity stress radiographs for the evaluation of supination-external rotation fibular fractures. J Bone Joint Surg Am 2007;89(5):994–999

Hoelsbrekken SE, Kaul-Jensen K, Mørch T, et al. Nonoperative treatment of the medial malleolus in bimalleolar and trimalleolar ankle fractures: a randomized controlled trial. J Orthop Trauma 2013;27(11):633–637

De Vries JS, Wijgman AJ, Sierevelt IN, Schaap GR. Long-term results of ankle fractures with a posterior malleolar fragment. J Foot Ankle Surg 2005;44(3):211–217

Gardner MJ, Brodsky A, Briggs SM, Nielson JH, Lorich DG. Fixation of posterior malleolar fractures provides greater syndesmotic stability. Clin Orthop Relat Res 2006;447(447):165–171

Chu A, Weiner L. Distal fibula malunions. J Am Acad Orthop Surg 2009;17(4):220–230

Marmor M, Kandemir U, Matityahu A, Jergesen H, McClellan T, Morshed S. A method for detection of lateral malleolar malrotation using conventional fluoroscopy. J Orthop Trauma 2013;27(12):e281–e284

Miller AN, Carroll EA, Parker RJ, Boraiah S, Helfet DL, Lorich DG. Direct visualization for syndesmotic stabilization of ankle fractures. Foot Ankle Int 2009;30(5):419–426

Summers HD, Sinclair MK, Stover MD. A reliable method for intraoperative evaluation of syndesmotic reduction. J Orthop Trauma 2013;27(4):196–200

Franke J, von Recum J, Suda AJ, Grützner PA, Wendl K. Intraoperative three-dimensional imaging in the treatment of acute unstable syndesmotic injuries. J Bone Joint Surg Am 2012;94(15):1386–1390

Park SS, Kubiak EN, Egol KA, Kummer F, Koval KJ. Stress radiographs after ankle fracture: the effect of ankle position and deltoid ligament status on medial clear space measurements. J Orthop Trauma 2006;20(1):11–18

Chapter 47: Talus Fractures

Dave Shearer, MD

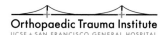

Orthopaedic Trauma Institute
UCSF + SAN FRANCISCO GENERAL HOSPITAL

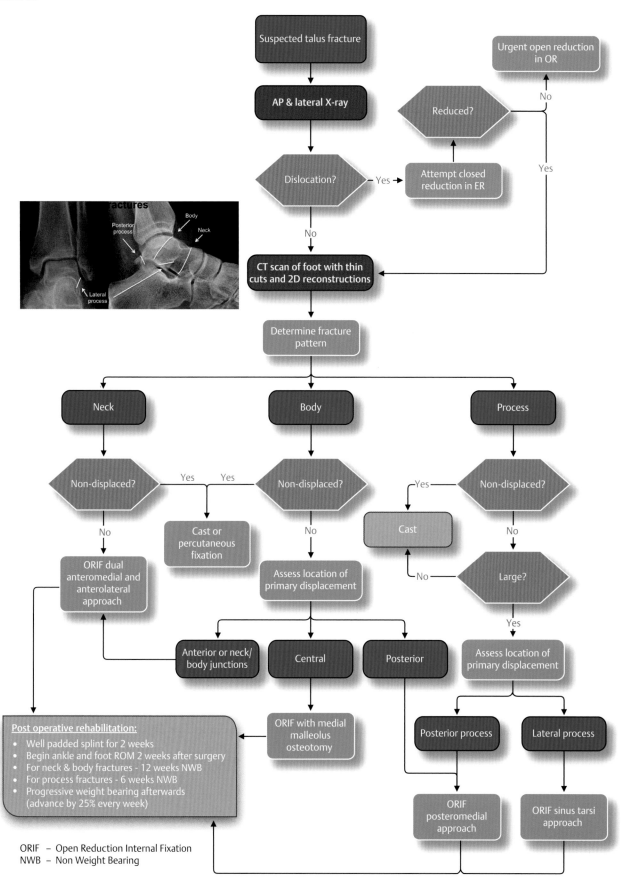

Suspected talus fracture

AP & lateral X-ray

Dislocation?

Yes → Attempt closed reduction in ER

Reduced?

No → Urgent open reduction in OR

Yes

No

CT scan of foot with thin cuts and 2D reconstructions

Determine fracture pattern

Neck | **Body** | **Process**

Non-displaced? (Neck) — Yes — Yes — Non-displaced? (Body)

No → ORIF dual anteromedial and anterolateral approach

Cast or percutaneous fixation

Non-displaced? (Process) — Yes → Cast

No

Large? — No → Cast

Non-displaced? (Body) — No → Assess location of primary displacement

Anterior or neck/body junctions | Central | Posterior

Large? — Yes → Assess location of primary displacement

ORIF with medial malleolus osteotomy

Posterior process | Lateral process

ORIF posteromedial approach

ORIF sinus tarsi approach

Post operative rehabilitation:
- Well padded splint for 2 weeks
- Begin ankle and foot ROM 2 weeks after surgery
- For neck & body fractures - 12 weeks NWB
- For process fractures - 6 weeks NWB
- Progressive weight bearing afterwards (advance by 25% every week)

ORIF – Open Reduction Internal Fixation
NWB – Non Weight Bearing

Suggested Readings

Vallier HA, Reichard SG, Boyd AJ, et al. A New Look at the Hawkins Classification for Talar Neck Fractures: Which Features of Injury and Treatment Are Predictive of Osteonecrosis? J Bone Joint Surg Am 2014;96(3):192–197

Hawkins LG. Fractures of the neck of the talus. J Bone Joint Surg Am 1970;52(5):991–1002

Lindvall E, Haidukewych G, DiPasquale T, et al. Open reduction and stable fixation of isolated, displaced talar neck and body fractures. J Bone Joint Surg Am 2004;86-A(10):2229–2234

Vallier HA, Nork SE, Benirschke SK, et al. Surgical treatment of talar body fractures. J Bone Joint Surg Am 2003;85-A(9):1716–1724

Vallier HA, Nork SE, Barei DP, Benirschke SK, Sangeorzan BJ. Talar neck fractures: results and outcomes. J Bone Joint Surg Am 2004;86-A(8):1616–1624

Chapter 48: Calcaneus Fractures

Richard Coughlin, MD, MSc

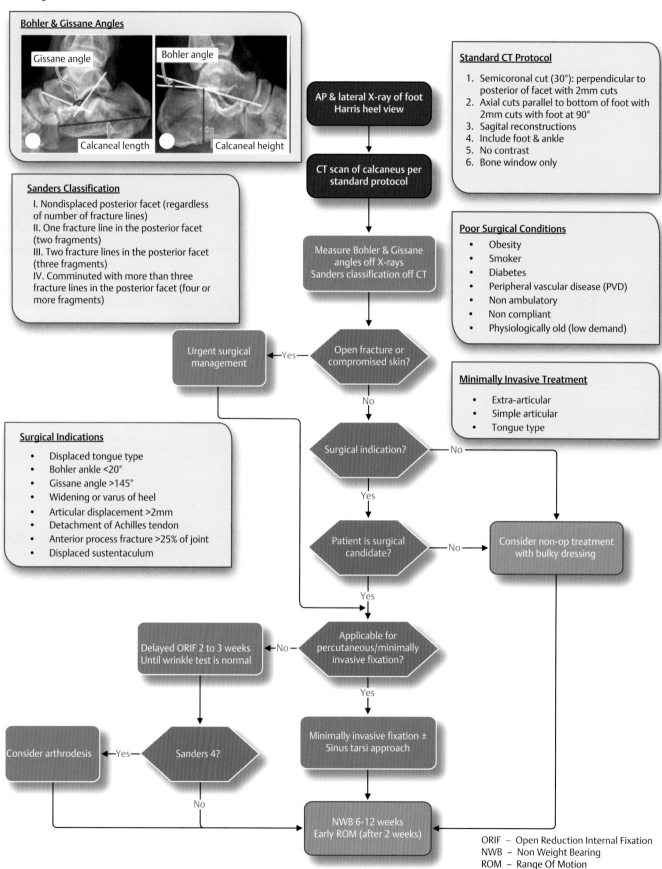

Bohler & Gissane Angles

Gissane angle

Bohler angle

Calcaneal length

Calcaneal height

Standard CT Protocol

1. Semicoronal cut (30°): perpendicular to posterior of facet with 2mm cuts
2. Axial cuts parallel to bottom of foot with 2mm cuts with foot at 90°
3. Sagital reconstructions
4. Include foot & ankle
5. No contrast
6. Bone window only

Sanders Classification

I. Nondisplaced posterior facet (regardless of number of fracture lines)
II. One fracture line in the posterior facet (two fragments)
III. Two fracture lines in the posterior facet (three fragments)
IV. Comminuted with more than three fracture lines in the posterior facet (four or more fragments)

Poor Surgical Conditions

- Obesity
- Smoker
- Diabetes
- Peripheral vascular disease (PVD)
- Non ambulatory
- Non compliant
- Physiologically old (low demand)

Minimally Invasive Treatment

- Extra-articular
- Simple articular
- Tongue type

Surgical Indications

- Displaced tongue type
- Bohler ankle <20°
- Gissane angle >145°
- Widening or varus of heel
- Articular displacement >2mm
- Detachment of Achilles tendon
- Anterior process fracture >25% of joint
- Displaced sustentaculum

AP & lateral X-ray of foot Harris heel view

CT scan of calcaneus per standard protocol

Measure Bohler & Gissane angles off X-rays Sanders classification off CT

Open fracture or compromised skin? —Yes→ Urgent surgical management

No

Surgical indication? —No→

Yes

Patient is surgical candidate? —No→ Consider non-op treatment with bulky dressing

Yes

Delayed ORIF 2 to 3 weeks Until wrinkle test is normal ←No— Applicable for percutaneous/minimally invasive fixation?

Yes

Consider arthrodesis ←Yes— Sanders 4?

No

Minimally invasive fixation ± Sinus tarsi approach

NWB 6-12 weeks Early ROM (after 2 weeks)

ORIF – Open Reduction Internal Fixation
NWB – Non Weight Bearing
ROM – Range Of Motion

Chapter 49: Lisfranc Fractures

Orthopaedic Trauma Institute
UCSF + SAN FRANCISCO GENERAL HOSPITAL

Dave Shearer, MD

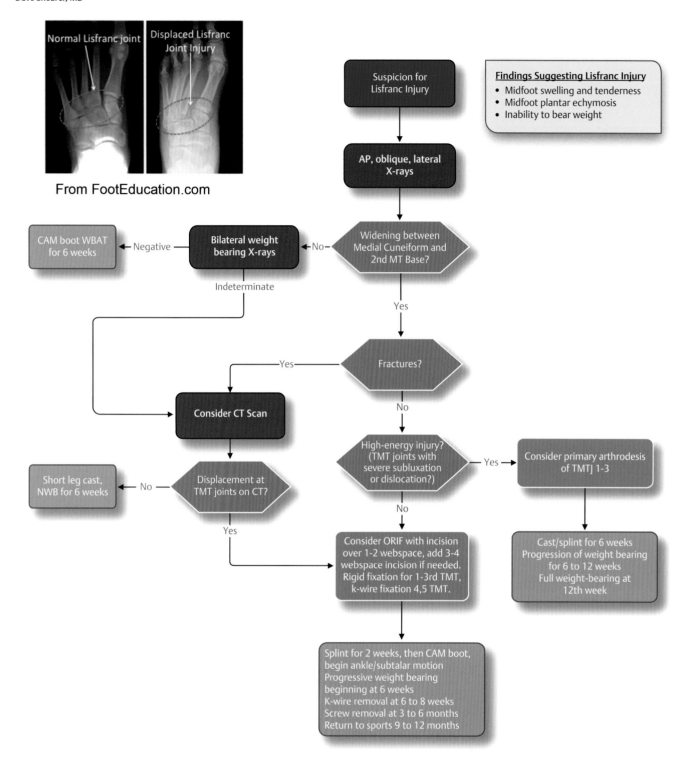

From FootEducation.com

Normal Lisfranc joint | Displaced Lisfranc Joint Injury

Findings Suggesting Lisfranc Injury
- Midfoot swelling and tenderness
- Midfoot plantar echymosis
- Inability to bear weight

Suspicion for Lisfranc Injury

AP, oblique, lateral X-rays

Widening between Medial Cuneiform and 2nd MT Base?

— No → Bilateral weight bearing X-rays — Negative → CAM boot WBAT for 6 weeks

Indeterminate

Yes

Fractures? — Yes →

No

Consider CT Scan

Displacement at TMT joints on CT? — No → Short leg cast, NWB for 6 weeks

Yes

High-energy injury? (TMT joints with severe subluxation or dislocation?) — Yes → Consider primary arthrodesis of TMTJ 1-3

No

Consider ORIF with incision over 1-2 webspace, add 3-4 webspace incision if needed. Rigid fixation for 1-3rd TMT, k-wire fixation 4,5 TMT.

Cast/splint for 6 weeks
Progression of weight bearing for 6 to 12 weeks
Full weight-bearing at 12th week

Splint for 2 weeks, then CAM boot, begin ankle/subtalar motion
Progressive weight bearing beginning at 6 weeks
K-wire removal at 6 to 8 weeks
Screw removal at 3 to 6 months
Return to sports 9 to 12 months

CAM   – Controlled Ankle Motion
NWB   – Non Weight Bearing
WBAT – Weight Bearing As Tolerated

Suggested Readings

Benirschke SK, Meinberg E, Anderson SA, Jones CB, Cole PA. Fractures and dislocations of the midfoot: Lisfranc and Chopart injuries. J Bone Joint Surg Am 2012;94(14):1325–1337

Scolaro J, Ahn J, Mehta S. Lisfranc fracture dislocations. Clin Orthop Relat Res 2011;469(7):2078–2080

Sherief TI, Mucci B, Greiss M. Lisfranc injury: how frequently does it get missed? And how can we improve? Injury 2007;38(7):856–860

Gupta RT, Wadhwa RP, Learch TJ, Herwick SM. Lisfranc injury: imaging findings for this important but often-missed diagnosis. Curr Probl Diagn Radiol 2008;37(3):115–126

Kaar S, Femino J, Morag Y. Lisfranc joint displacement following sequential ligament sectioning. J Bone Joint Surg Am 2007;89(10):2225–2232

Henning JA, Jones CB, Sietsema DL, Bohay DR, Anderson JG. Open reduction internal fixation versus primary arthrodesis for lisfranc injuries: a prospective randomized study. Foot Ankle Int 2009;30(10):913–922

Raikin SM, Elias I, Dheer S, Besser MP, Morrison WB, Zoga AC. Prediction of midfoot instability in the subtle Lisfranc injury. Comparison of magnetic resonance imaging with intraoperative findings. J Bone Joint Surg Am 2009;91(4):892–899

Kadow TR, Siska PA, Evans AR, Sands SS, Tarkin IS. Staged treatment of high energy midfoot fracture dislocations. Foot Ankle Int 2014;35(12):1287–1291

Faciszewski T, Burks RT, Manaster BJ. Subtle injuries of the Lisfranc joint. J Bone Joint Surg Am 1990;72(10):1519–1522

Coetzee JC, Ly TV. Treatment of primarily ligamentous Lisfranc joint injuries: primary arthrodesis compared with open reduction and internal fixation. Surgical technique. J Bone Joint Surg Am 2007; 89(2, Suppl 2 Pt.1):122–127

Rammelt S, Schneiders W, Schikore H, Holch M, Heineck J, Zwipp H. Primary open reduction and fixation compared with delayed corrective arthrodesis in the treatment of tarsometatarsal (Lisfranc) fracture dislocation. J Bone Joint Surg Br 2008;90(11):1499–1506

Dave Shearer, MD

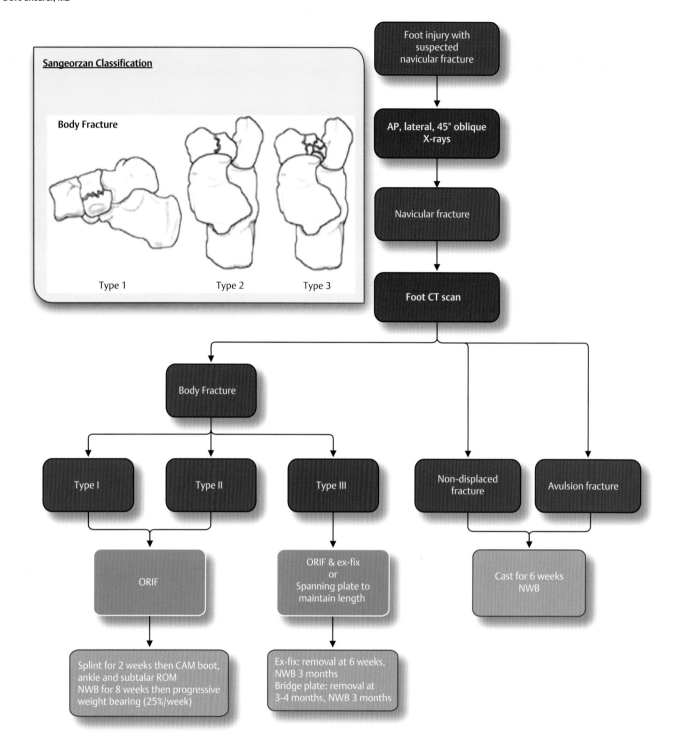

Sangeorzan Classification

Body Fracture

Type 1   Type 2   Type 3

Foot injury with suspected navicular fracture

AP, lateral, 45° oblique X-rays

Navicular fracture

Foot CT scan

Body Fracture

Type I   Type II   Type III

Non-displaced fracture

Avulsion fracture

ORIF

ORIF & ex-fix
or
Spanning plate to maintain length

Cast for 6 weeks NWB

Splint for 2 weeks then CAM boot, ankle and subtalar ROM
NWB for 8 weeks then progressive weight bearing (25%/week)

Ex-fix: removal at 6 weeks, NWB 3 months
Bridge plate: removal at 3-4 months, NWB 3 months

Ex-Fix – External Fixator
NWB   – Non Weight Bearing
ORIF   – Open Reduction Internal Fixation

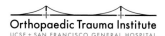

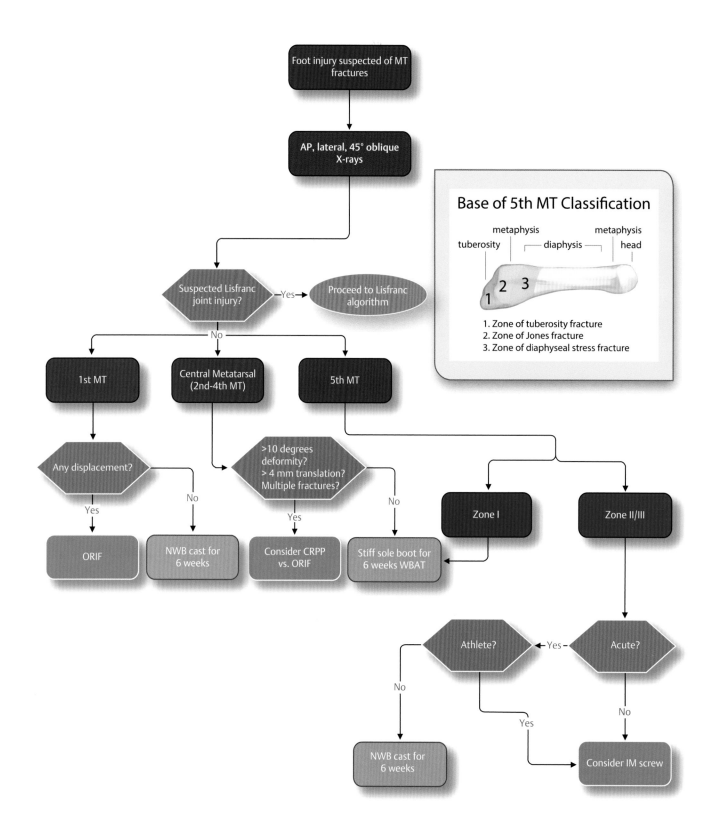

Base of 5th MT Classification

tuberosity · metaphysis · diaphysis · metaphysis · head

1. Zone of tuberosity fracture
2. Zone of Jones fracture
3. Zone of diaphyseal stress fracture

Foot injury suspected of MT fractures
↓
AP, lateral, 45° oblique X-rays
↓
Suspected Lisfranc joint injury? — Yes → Proceed to Lisfranc algorithm
↓ No

- **1st MT**
  - Any displacement?
    - Yes → ORIF
    - No → NWB cast for 6 weeks
- **Central Metatarsal (2nd-4th MT)**
  - >10 degrees deformity? > 4 mm translation? Multiple fractures?
    - Yes → Consider CRPP vs. ORIF
    - No → Stiff sole boot for 6 weeks WBAT
- **5th MT**
  - Zone I → Stiff sole boot for 6 weeks WBAT
  - Zone II/III
    - Acute?
      - Yes → Athlete?
        - No → NWB cast for 6 weeks
        - Yes → Consider IM screw
      - No → Consider IM screw

Suggested Readings

Torg JS, Balduini FC, Zelko RR, Pavlov H, Peff TC, Das M. Fractures of the base of the fifth metatarsal distal to the tuberosity. Classification and guidelines for non-surgical and surgical management. J Bone Joint Surg Am 1984;66(2):209–214

Shereff MJ. Fractures of the forefoot. Instr Course Lect 1990;39:133–140

Armagan OE, Shereff MJ. Injuries to the toes and metatarsals. Orthop Clin North Am 2001;32(1):1–10

Coughlin MJ, Saltzman CL, Anderson RB, et al. Mann's surgery of the foot and ankle. Vol. 1. Philadelphia: Saunders/Elsevier; 2014

Dave Shearer, MD

Orthopaedic Trauma Institute
UCSF + SAN FRANCISCO GENERAL HOSPITAL

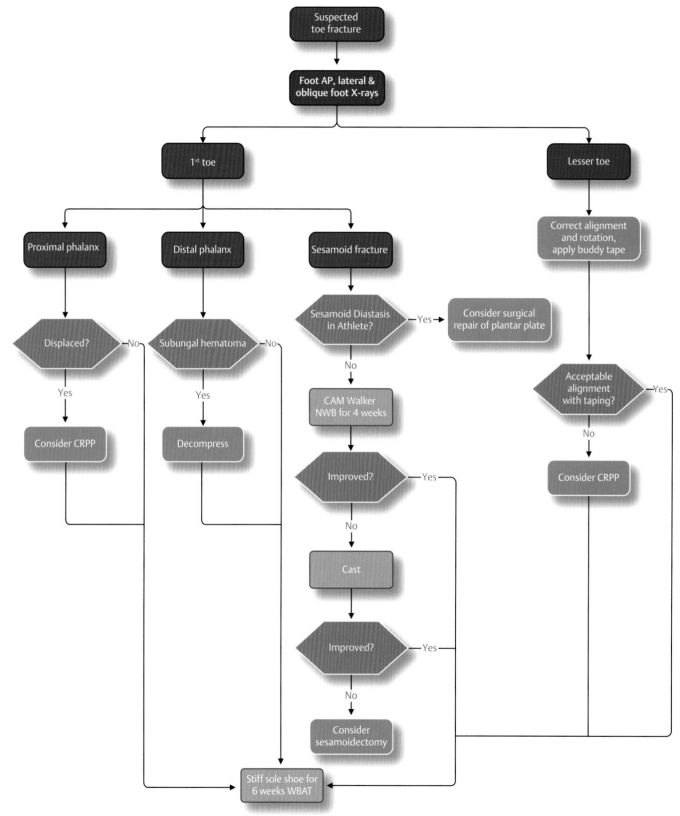

CAM – Controlled Ankle Motion
CRPP – Closed Reduction Percutaneous Pinning
NWB – Non Weight Bearing
WBAT – Weight Bearing As Tolerated

Suggested Readings

Coughlin MJ, Saltzman CL, Anderson RB, et al. Mann's surgery of the foot and ankle. Vol. 1 Vol. 1. Philadelphia: Saunders/ Elsevier; 2014.

Jahss MH. Stubbing injuries to the hallux. Foot Ankle. 1981 May;1(6):327–332.

McCormick JJ, Anderson RB. The Great Toe: Failed Turf Toe, Chronic Turf Toe, and Complicated Sesamoid Injuries. Foot and Ankle Clinics. 2009 Jun;14(2):135–150.

Chapter 53: Pelvic Ring Fractures

Amir Matityahu, MD

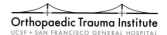
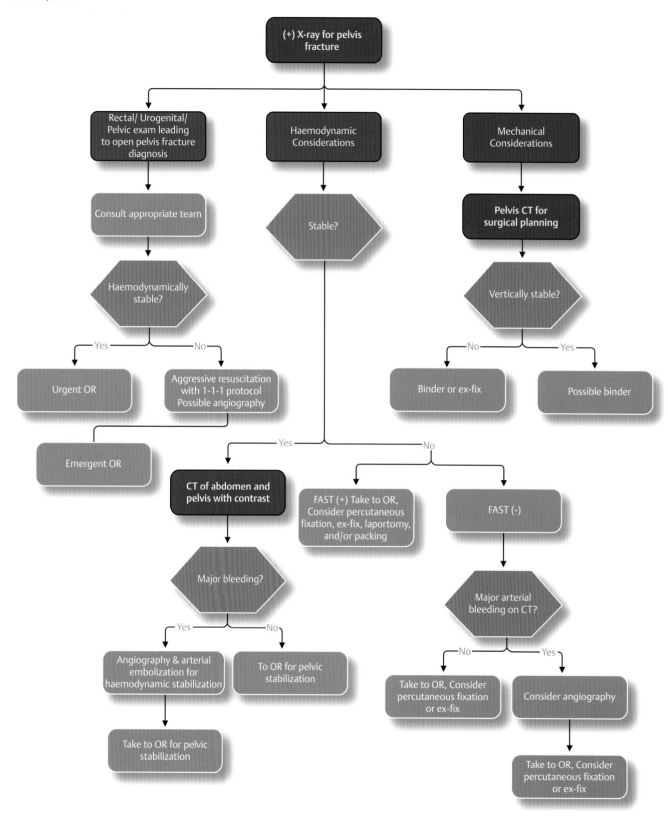

FAST - Focused Assessment with Sonography in Trauma

Suggested Readings

DeAngelis NA, Wixted JJ, Drew J, Eskander MS, Eskander JP, French BG. Use of the trauma pelvic orthotic device (T-POD) for provisional stabilisation of anterior-posterior compression type pelvic fractures: a cadaveric study. Injury 2008;39(8):903–906

White CE, Hsu JR, Holcomb JB. Haemodynamically unstable pelvic fractures. Injury 2009;40(10):1023–1030

Grotz MR, Allami MK, Harwood P, Pape HC, Krettek C, Giannoudis PV. Open pelvic fractures: epidemiology, current concepts of management and outcome. Injury 2005;36(1):1–13

Chapter 54: Acetabulum Fractures

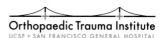

Amir Matityahu, MD

Lateral View of Pelvis

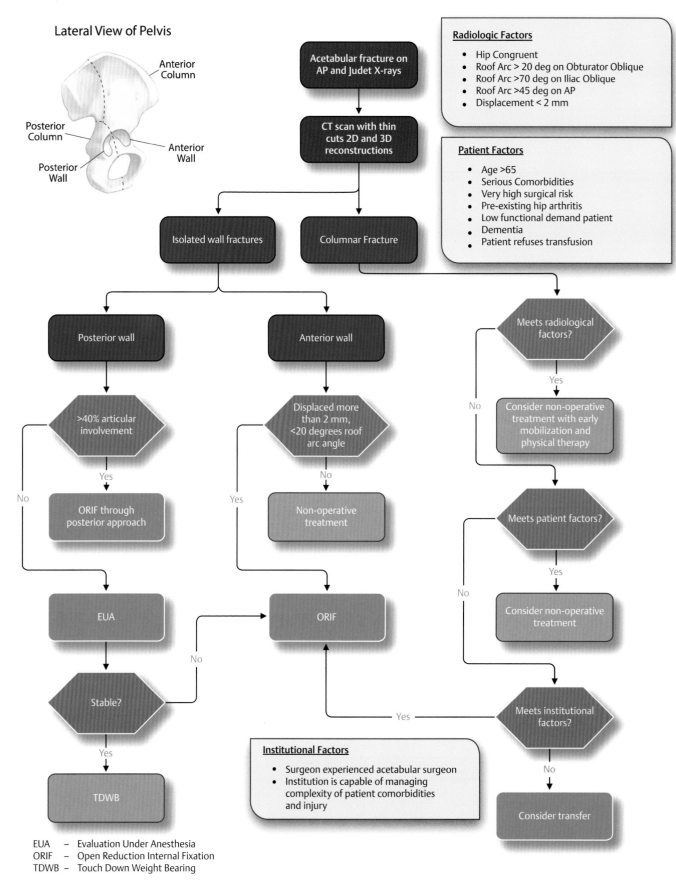

Radiologic Factors

- Hip Congruent
- Roof Arc > 20 deg on Obturator Oblique
- Roof Arc >70 deg on Iliac Oblique
- Roof Arc >45 deg on AP
- Displacement < 2 mm

Patient Factors

- Age >65
- Serious Comorbidities
- Very high surgical risk
- Pre-existing hip arthritis
- Low functional demand patient
- Dementia
- Patient refuses transfusion

Institutional Factors

- Surgeon experienced acetabular surgeon
- Institution is capable of managing complexity of patient comorbidities and injury

Acetabular fracture on AP and Judet X-rays

CT scan with thin cuts 2D and 3D reconstructions

Isolated wall fractures

Columnar Fracture

Posterior wall

Anterior wall

Meets radiological factors?

>40% articular involvement

Displaced more than 2 mm, <20 degrees roof arc angle

Consider non-operative treatment with early mobilization and physical therapy

ORIF through posterior approach

Non-operative treatment

Meets patient factors?

EUA

ORIF

Consider non-operative treatment

Stable?

Meets institutional factors?

TDWB

Consider transfer

EUA – Evaluation Under Anesthesia
ORIF – Open Reduction Internal Fixation
TDWB – Touch Down Weight Bearing

Suggested Readings

Tornetta P III. Non-operative management of acetabular fractures. The use of dynamic stress views. J Bone Joint Surg Br 1999;81(1):67–70

Vrahas MS, Widding KK, Thomas KA. The effects of simulated transverse, anterior column, and posterior column fractures of the acetabulum on the stability of the hip joint. J Bone Joint Surg Am 1999;81(7):966–974

Amir Matityahu, MD

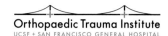

Orthopaedic Trauma Institute
UCSF + SAN FRANCISCO GENERAL HOSPITAL

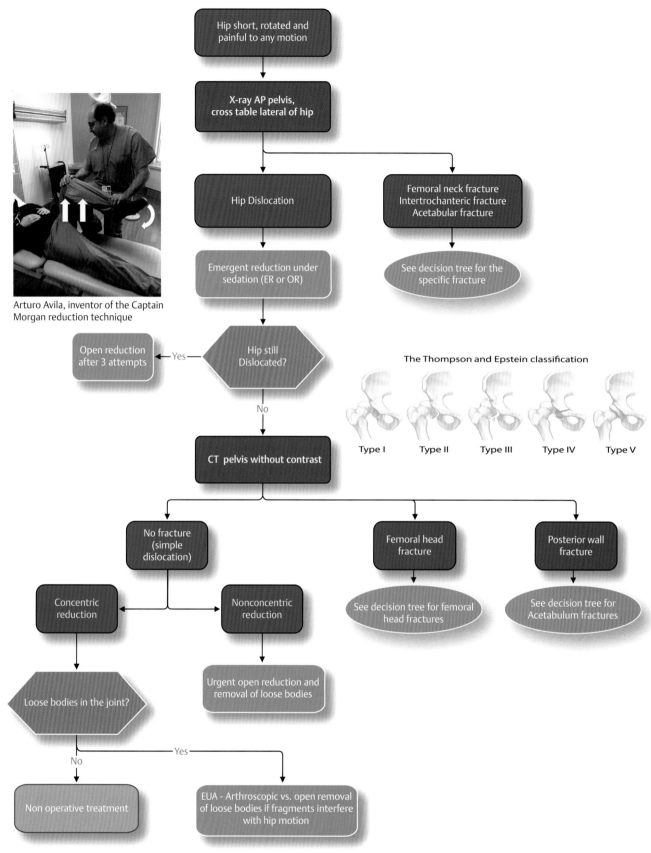

Arturo Avila, inventor of the Captain Morgan reduction technique

Hip short, rotated and painful to any motion

X-ray AP pelvis, cross table lateral of hip

Hip Dislocation

Femoral neck fracture Intertrochanteric fracture Acetabular fracture

Emergent reduction under sedation (ER or OR)

See decision tree for the specific fracture

Hip still Dislocated?

Open reduction after 3 attempts ← Yes

No

CT pelvis without contrast

The Thompson and Epstein classification

Type I   Type II   Type III   Type IV   Type V

No fracture (simple dislocation)

Femoral head fracture

Posterior wall fracture

See decision tree for femoral head fractures

See decision tree for Acetabulum fractures

Concentric reduction

Nonconcentric reduction

Loose bodies in the joint?

Urgent open reduction and removal of loose bodies

No   Yes

Non operative treatment

EUA - Arthroscopic vs. open removal of loose bodies if fragments interfere with hip motion

EUA – Evaluation Under Anesthesia

Suggested Readings

Hendey GW, Avila A. The Captain Morgan technique for the reduction of the dislocated hip. Annals of emergency medicine. 2011 Dec 31;58(6):536-40.

Chapter 56: Femoral Head Fractures

Amir Matityahu, MD

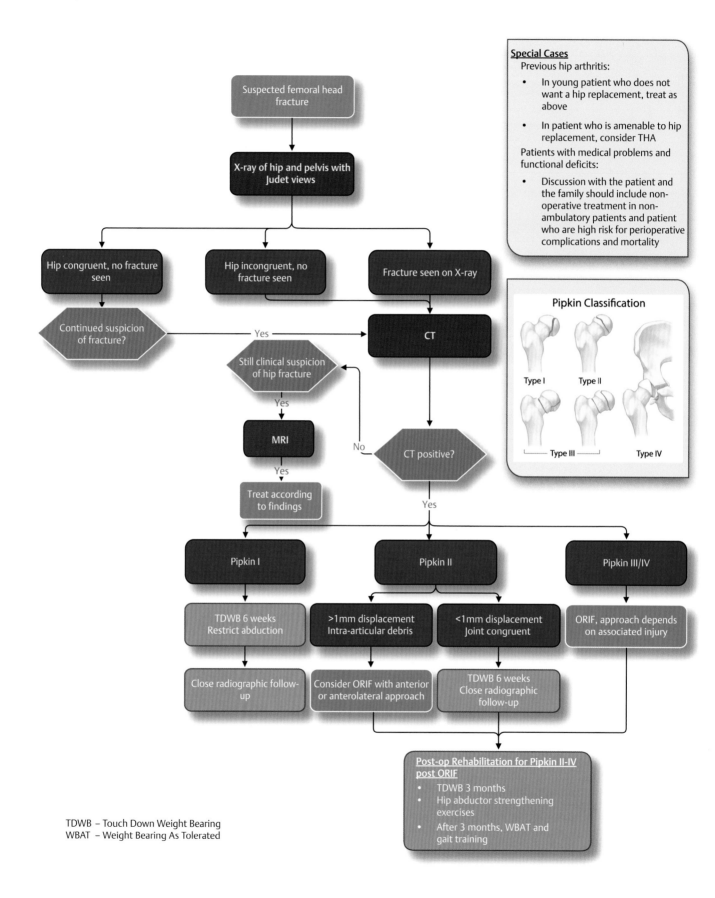

Special Cases
Previous hip arthritis:

- In young patient who does not want a hip replacement, treat as above

- In patient who is amenable to hip replacement, consider THA

Patients with medical problems and functional deficits:

- Discussion with the patient and the family should include non-operative treatment in non-ambulatory patients and patient who are high risk for perioperative complications and mortality

Suspected femoral head fracture

X-ray of hip and pelvis with Judet views

Hip congruent, no fracture seen

Hip incongruent, no fracture seen

Fracture seen on X-ray

Continued suspicion of fracture?

Still clinical suspicion of hip fracture

CT

MRI

CT positive?

Treat according to findings

Pipkin Classification

Type I   Type II

Type III   Type IV

Pipkin I

Pipkin II

Pipkin III/IV

TDWB 6 weeks
Restrict abduction

>1mm displacement
Intra-articular debris

<1mm displacement
Joint congruent

ORIF, approach depends on associated injury

Close radiographic follow-up

Consider ORIF with anterior or anterolateral approach

TDWB 6 weeks
Close radiographic follow-up

Post-op Rehabilitation for Pipkin II-IV post ORIF
- TDWB 3 months
- Hip abductor strengthening exercises
- After 3 months, WBAT and gait training

TDWB – Touch Down Weight Bearing
WBAT – Weight Bearing As Tolerated

Chapter 57: Femoral Intertrochanteric Fractures

Dave Shearer, MD

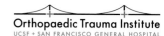
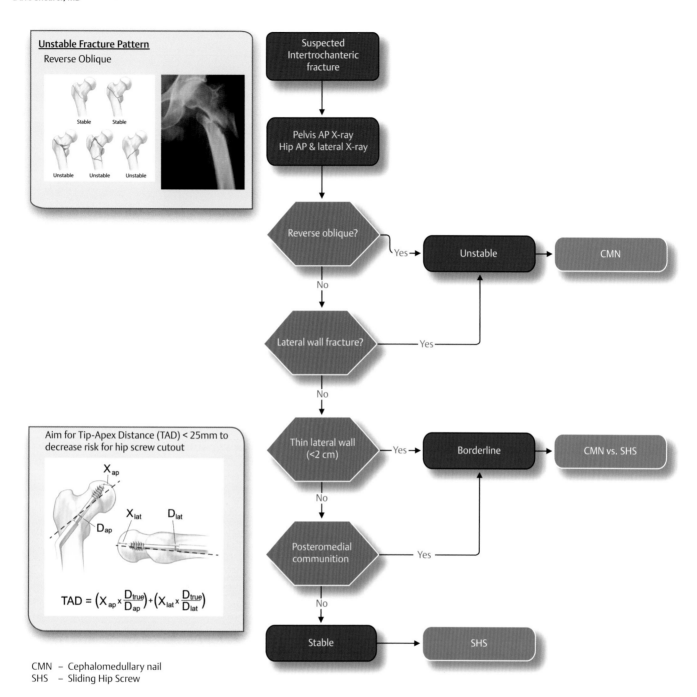

CMN – Cephalomedullary nail
SHS – Sliding Hip Screw

Eric Meinberg, MD

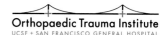

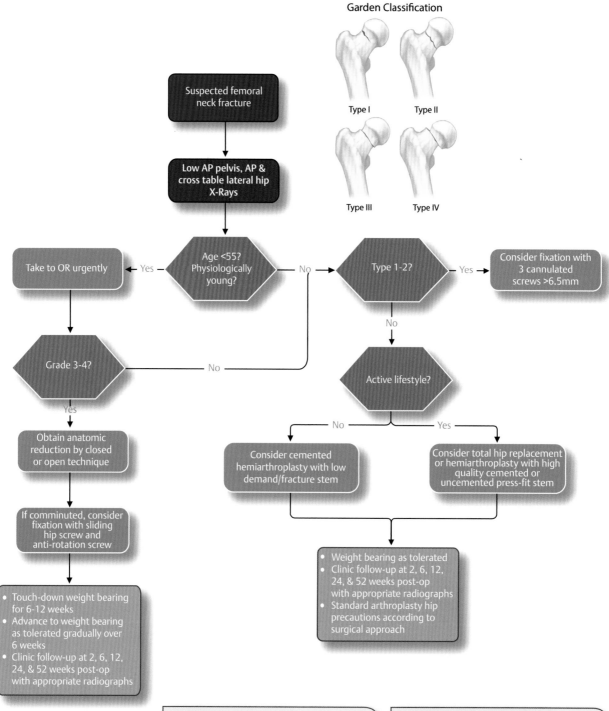

Garden Classification

Type I Type II

Type III Type IV

Suspected femoral neck fracture

Low AP pelvis, AP & cross table lateral hip X-Rays

Age <55? Physiologically young?

Take to OR urgently ←Yes

No→ Type 1-2? Yes→ Consider fixation with 3 cannulated screws >6.5mm

No

Grade 3-4? —No—

Active lifestyle?

Yes↓

Obtain anatomic reduction by closed or open technique

No→ Consider cemented hemiarthroplasty with low demand/fracture stem

Yes→ Consider total hip replacement or hemiarthroplasty with high quality cemented or uncemented press-fit stem

If comminuted, consider fixation with sliding hip screw and anti-rotation screw

- Weight bearing as tolerated
- Clinic follow-up at 2, 6, 12, 24, & 52 weeks post-op with appropriate radiographs
- Standard arthroplasty hip precautions according to surgical approach

- Touch-down weight bearing for 6-12 weeks
- Advance to weight bearing as tolerated gradually over 6 weeks
- Clinic follow-up at 2, 6, 12, 24, & 52 weeks post-op with appropriate radiographs

Definition of Active Lifestyle
One of the following:
- Active >8 hours per day
- Regular physical activity
- No assistive device for ambulation
- Independent in all ADLs

Definition of Physiologically Young
No history of the following:
- CHF
- CVA
- Type II diabetes requiring insulin
- Creatinine >2
- Medical co-morbidities are stable and do not impact ADLs

ADL – Activity of Daily Living
CHF – Congestive Heart Failure
CVA – Cerebrovascular Accident

Suggested Readings

Barnes R, Brown JT, Garden RS, Nicoll EA. Subcapital fractures of the femur. A prospective review. J Bone Joint Surg Br 1976;58(1):2–24

Blomfeldt R, Törnkvist H, Eriksson K, Söderqvist A, Ponzer S, Tidermark J. A randomised controlled trial comparing bipolar hemiarthroplasty with total hip replacement for displaced intracapsular fractures of the femoral neck in elderly patients. J Bone Joint Surg Br 2007;89(2):160–165

Evaniew N, Madden K, Bhandari M. Cochrane in CORR®: Arthroplasties (with and without bone cement) for proximal femoral fractures in adults. Clin Orthop Relat Res 2014;472(5):1367–1372

Dave Shearer, MD

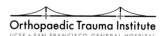

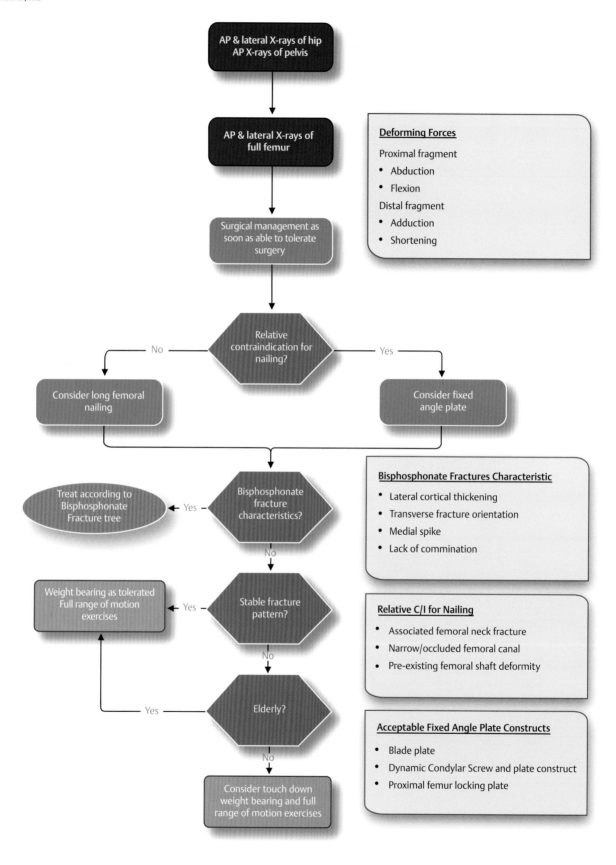

Deforming Forces

Proximal fragment
- Abduction
- Flexion

Distal fragment
- Adduction
- Shortening

Bisphosphonate Fractures Characteristic
- Lateral cortical thickening
- Transverse fracture orientation
- Medial spike
- Lack of commination

Relative C/I for Nailing
- Associated femoral neck fracture
- Narrow/occluded femoral canal
- Pre-existing femoral shaft deformity

Acceptable Fixed Angle Plate Constructs
- Blade plate
- Dynamic Condylar Screw and plate construct
- Proximal femur locking plate

Chapter 60: Spinal Cord Injury (SCI)

Jeremie Larouche, MD and R. Trigg McClellan, MD

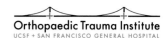

Orthopaedic Trauma Institute
UCSF + SAN FRANCISCO GENERAL HOSPITAL

ASIA Impairment Scale

A	Complete	No sensory or motor function is preserved in sacral segments S4-S5.
B	Incomplete	Sensory, but not motor, function is preserved below neurologic level and extends through sacral segments S4-S5.
C	Incomplete	Motor function is preserved below the neurologic level, and most key muscles below the neurologic level have muscle grade less than 3.
D	Incomplete	Motor function is preserved below the neurologic level, and most key muscles below the neurologic level have muscle grade greater than or equal to 3
E	Normal	Sensory and motor functions are normal

Note: ASIA grade E is used to identify an individual which temporarily had a neurological deficit but has since regained normal sensory and motor function

Spinal Cord Syndromes

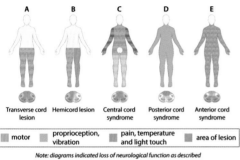

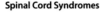

A	B	C	D	E
Transverse cord lesion	Hemicord lesion	Central cord syndrome	Posterior cord syndrome	Anterior cord syndrome

■ motor ■ proprioception, vibration ■ pain, temperature and light touch ■ area of lesion

Note: diagrams indicated loss of neurological function as described

Definitions

Spinal Shock: Loss of motor and sensation below a level of injury associated with initial areflexia/hyporeflexia. Over the course of a few days, reflexes return and become hyperreflexic.

Neogenic shock: Loss of sympathetic drive to the cardiovascular system with spinal cord injuries normally at the level of T6 or above. Manifested with:
> Bradycardia
> Hypotension

SCI Complications

- Pressure ulcers
- Deep vein thrombosis (DVT)
- Urosepsis
- Bradycardia
- Orthostatic hypotension
- Autonomic dysreflexia
- Depression

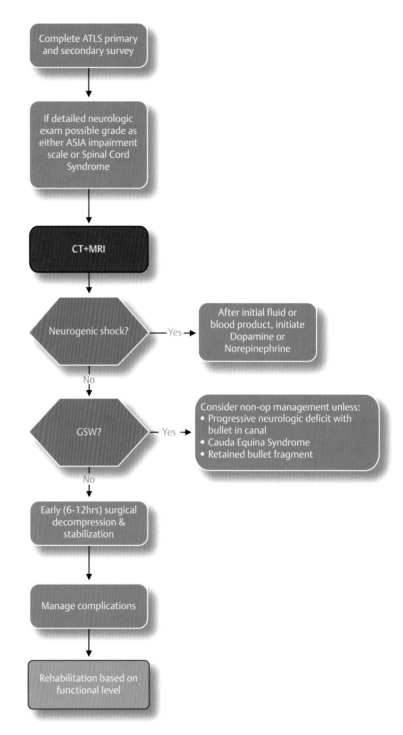

Complete ATLS primary and secondary survey

↓

If detailed neurologic exam possible grade as either ASIA impairment scale or Spinal Cord Syndrome

↓

CT+MRI

↓

Neurogenic shock? —Yes→ After initial fluid or blood product, initiate Dopamine or Norepinephrine

No
↓

GSW? —Yes→ Consider non-op management unless:
- Progressive neurologic deficit with bullet in canal
- Cauda Equina Syndrome
- Retained bullet fragment

No
↓

Early (6-12hrs) surgical decompression & stabilization

↓

Manage complications

↓

Rehabilitation based on functional level

ASIA – American Spinal Injury Association
ATLS – Advanced Trauma Life Support
GSW – Gun Shot Wound

Suggested Readings

ATLS Subcommittee; American College of Surgeons' Committee on Trauma; International ATLS working group. Advanced trauma life support (ATLS®): the ninth edition. J Trauma Acute Care Surg 2013;74(5):1363–1366

Chapter 61: Adult C-Spine Clearance After Blunt Trauma

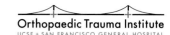

Jeremie Larouche, MD and R. Trigg McClellan, MD

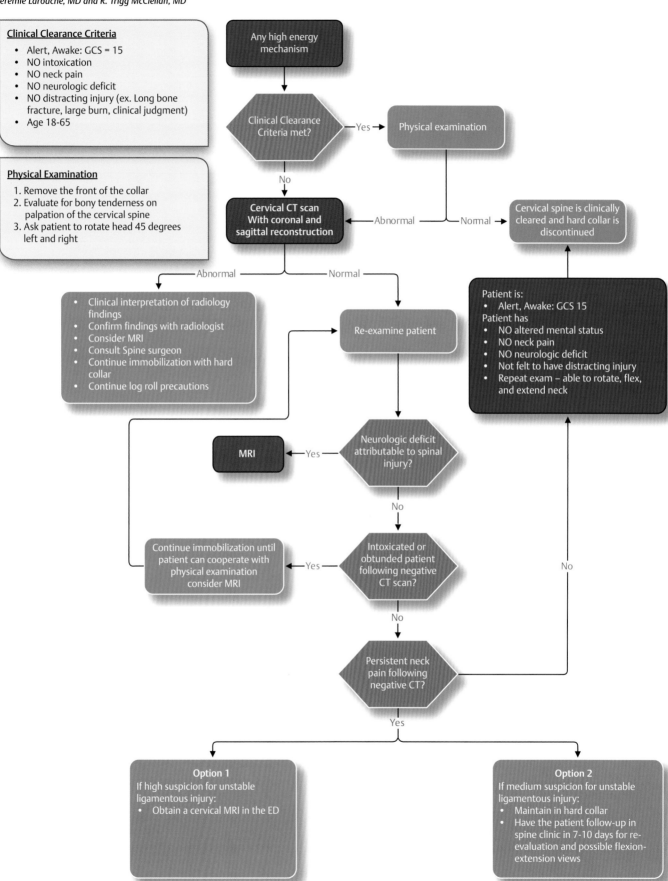

Clinical Clearance Criteria
- Alert, Awake: GCS = 15
- NO intoxication
- NO neck pain
- NO neurologic deficit
- NO distracting injury (ex. Long bone fracture, large burn, clinical judgment)
- Age 18-65

Physical Examination
1. Remove the front of the collar
2. Evaluate for bony tenderness on palpation of the cervical spine
3. Ask patient to rotate head 45 degrees left and right

Any high energy mechanism

Clinical Clearance Criteria met?

Yes → Physical examination

No

Cervical CT scan With coronal and sagittal reconstruction ← Abnormal ← Normal → Cervical spine is clinically cleared and hard collar is discontinued

Abnormal — Normal

- Clinical interpretation of radiology findings
- Confirm findings with radiologist
- Consider MRI
- Consult Spine surgeon
- Continue immobilization with hard collar
- Continue log roll precautions

Re-examine patient

Patient is:
- Alert, Awake: GCS 15
Patient has
- NO altered mental status
- NO neck pain
- NO neurologic deficit
- Not felt to have distracting injury
- Repeat exam – able to rotate, flex, and extend neck

MRI ← Yes — Neurologic deficit attributable to spinal injury?

No

Continue immobilization until patient can cooperate with physical examination consider MRI ← Yes — Intoxicated or obtunded patient following negative CT scan?

No

No

Persistent neck pain following negative CT?

Yes

Option 1
If high suspicion for unstable ligamentous injury:
- Obtain a cervical MRI in the ED

Option 2
If medium suspicion for unstable ligamentous injury:
- Maintain in hard collar
- Have the patient follow-up in spine clinic in 7-10 days for re-evaluation and possible flexion-extension views

Suggested Readings

Hoffman JR, Mower WR, Wolfson AB, Todd KH, Zucker MI; National Emergency X-Radiography Utilization Study Group. Validity of a set of clinical criteria to rule out injury to the cervical spine in patients with blunt trauma. N Engl J Med 2000;343(2):94–99

Gebauer G, Osterman M, Harrop J, Vaccaro A. Spinal cord injury resulting from injury missed on CT scan: the danger of relying on CT alone for collar removal. Clin Orthop Relat Res 2012;470(6):1652–1657

Badhiwala JH, Lai CK, Alhazzani W, et al. Cervical spine clearance in obtunded patients after blunt traumatic injury: a systematic review. Ann Intern Med 2015;162(6):429–437

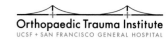
Orthopaedic Trauma Institute
UCSF + SAN FRANCISCO GENERAL HOSPITAL

Jeremie Larouche, MD and R. Trigg McClellan, MD

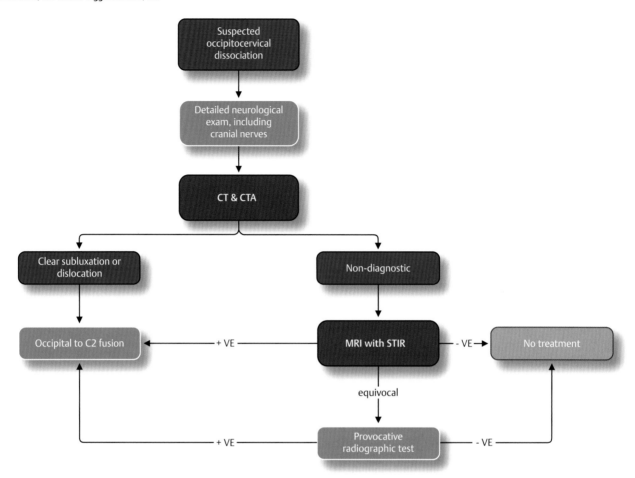

CTA – CT Angio
STIR – Short Tau Inversion Recovery

Suggested Readings

Kasliwal MK, Fontes RB, Traynelis VC. Occipitocervical dissociation-incidence, evaluation, and treatment. Curr Rev Musculoskelet Med 2016;9(3):247–254

Child Z, Rau D, Lee MJ, et al. The provocative radiographic traction test for diagnosing craniocervical dissociation: a cadaveric biomechanical study and reappraisal of the pathogenesis of instability. Spine J 2016;16(9):1116–1123

Jeremie Larouche, MD and R. Trigg McClellan, MD

Orthopaedic Trauma Institute
UCSF + SAN FRANCISCO GENERAL HOSPITAL

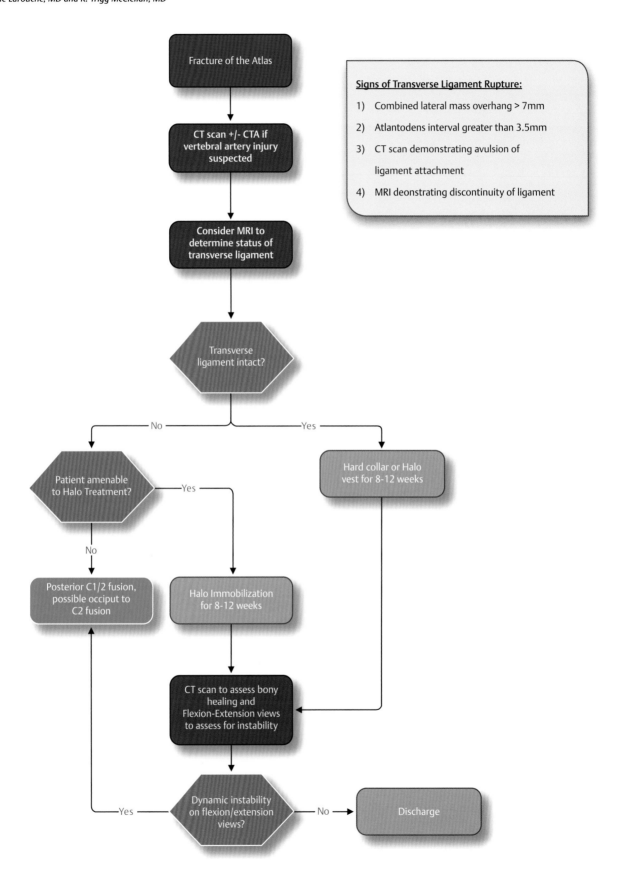

Fracture of the Atlas

CT scan +/- CTA if vertebral artery injury suspected

Consider MRI to determine status of transverse ligament

Transverse ligament intact?

Signs of Transverse Ligament Rupture:

1) Combined lateral mass overhang > 7mm

2) Atlantodens interval greater than 3.5mm

3) CT scan demonstrating avulsion of ligament attachment

4) MRI deonstrating discontinuity of ligament

No — Patient amenable to Halo Treatment?

Yes — Hard collar or Halo vest for 8-12 weeks

Yes — Halo Immobilization for 8-12 weeks

No — Posterior C1/2 fusion, possible occiput to C2 fusion

CT scan to assess bony healing and Flexion-Extension views to assess for instability

Dynamic instability on flexion/extension views?

Yes

No → Discharge

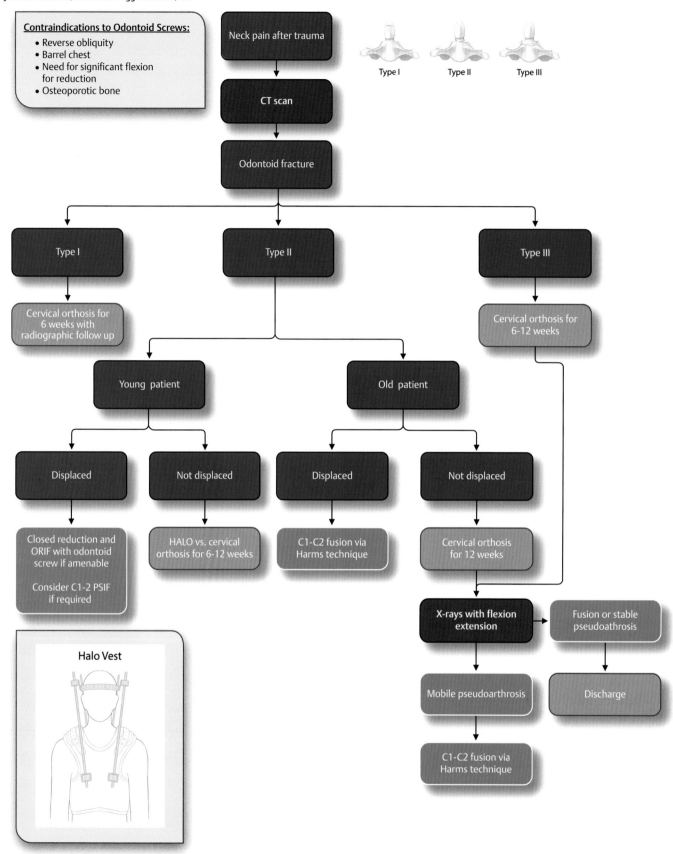

Jeremie Larouche, MD and R. Trigg McClellan, MD

Orthopaedic Trauma Institute
UCSF + SAN FRANCISCO GENERAL HOSPITAL

Contraindications to Odontoid Screws:
- Reverse obliquity
- Barrel chest
- Need for significant flexion for reduction
- Osteoporotic bone

Neck pain after trauma

CT scan

Odontoid fracture

Type I   Type II   Type III

Type I

Type II

Type III

Cervical orthosis for 6 weeks with radiographic follow up

Cervical orthosis for 6-12 weeks

Young patient

Old patient

Displaced

Not displaced

Displaced

Not displaced

Closed reduction and ORIF with odontoid screw if amenable

Consider C1-2 PSIF if required

HALO vs. cervical orthosis for 6-12 weeks

C1-C2 fusion via Harms technique

Cervical orthosis for 12 weeks

X-rays with flexion extension

Fusion or stable pseudoathrosis

Mobile pseudoarthrosis

Discharge

C1-C2 fusion via Harms technique

Halo Vest

Chapter 65: C2 Traumatic Spondylolisthesis

Jeremie Larouche, MD and R. Trigg McClellan, MD

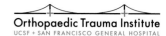

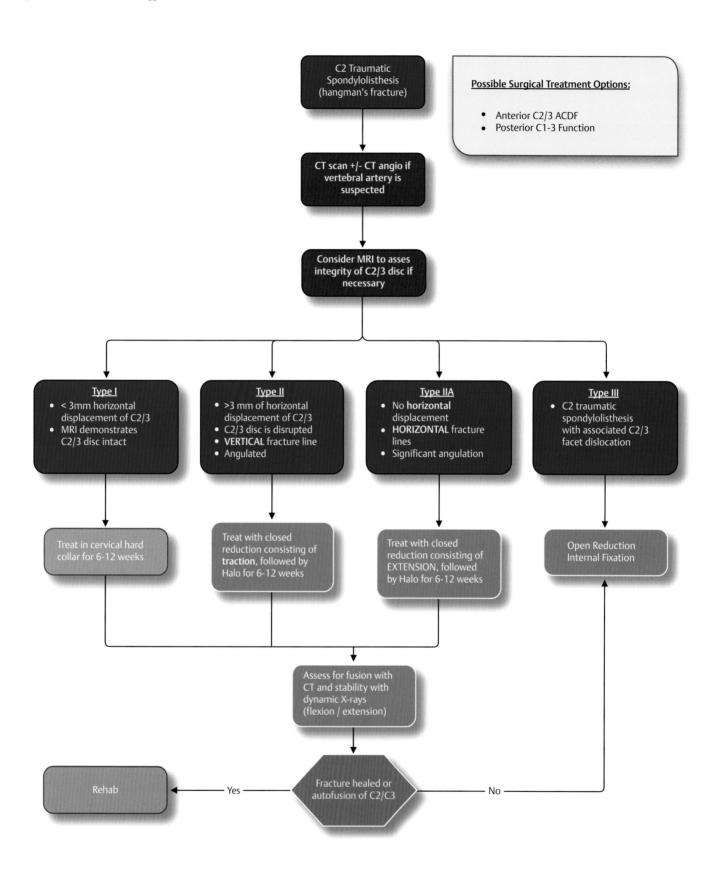

Chapter 66: C3-C7 Facet Dislocations

Jeremie Larouche, MD and R. Trigg McClellan, MD

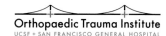

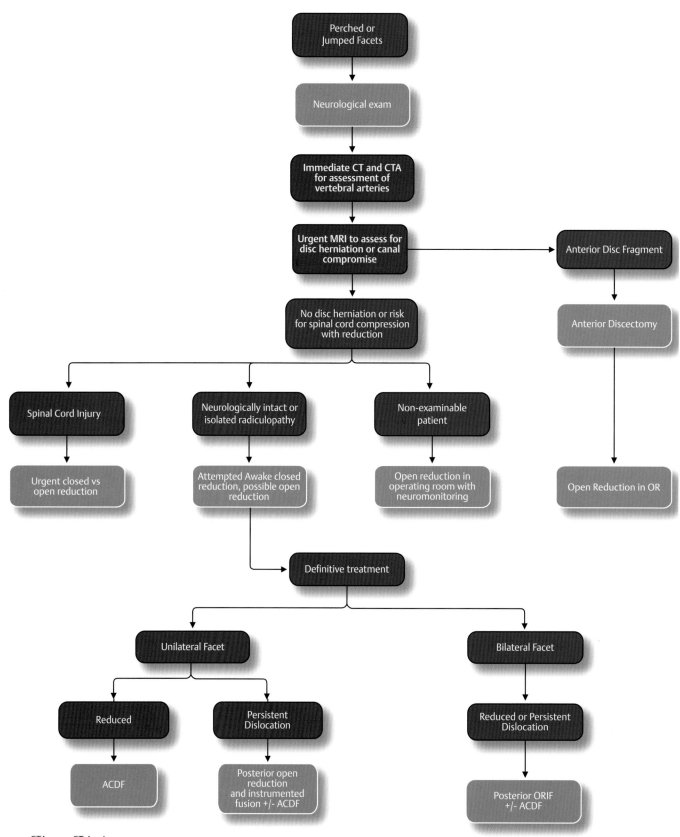

CTA – CT Angio
ACDF – Anterior Cervical Discectomy and Fusion
ORIF – Open Reduction Internal Fixation

Chapter 67: C3-C7 Lateral Mass Fractures

Jeremie Larouche, MD and R. Trigg McClellan, MD

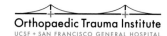
Orthopaedic Trauma Institute
UCSF + SAN FRANCISCO GENERAL HOSPITAL

Lateral Mass Fracture

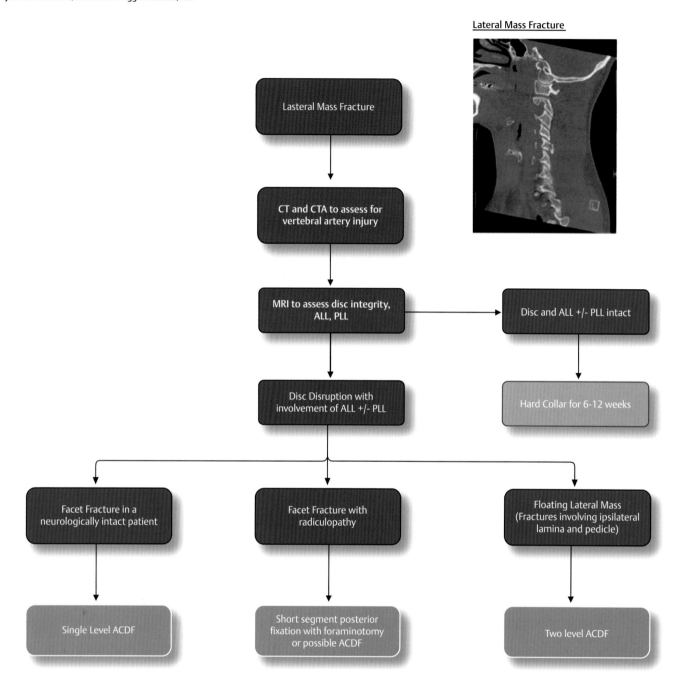

ACDF – Anterior Cervical Discectomy and Fusion
CTA – CT Angio
ALL – Anterior Longitudinal Ligament
PLL – Posterior Longitudinal Ligament

Suggested Readings

Aarabi B, Mirvis S, Shanmuganathan K, et al. Comparative effectiveness of surgical versus nonoperative management of unilateral, nondisplaced, subaxial cervical spine facet fractures without evidence of spinal cord injury: clinical article. J Neurosurg Spine 2014;20(3):270–277

Kepler CK, Vaccaro AR, Chen E, et al. Treatment of isolated cervical facet fractures: a systematic review. J Neurosurg Spine 2015;24(2):1–8

Manoso MW, Moore TA, Agel J, Bellabarba C, Bransford RJ. Floating Lateral Mass Fractures of the Cervical Spine. Spine 2016;41(18):1421–1427

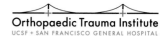

Orthopaedic Trauma Institute
UCSF + SAN FRANCISCO GENERAL HOSPITAL

Jeremie Larouche, MD and R. Trigg McClellan, MD

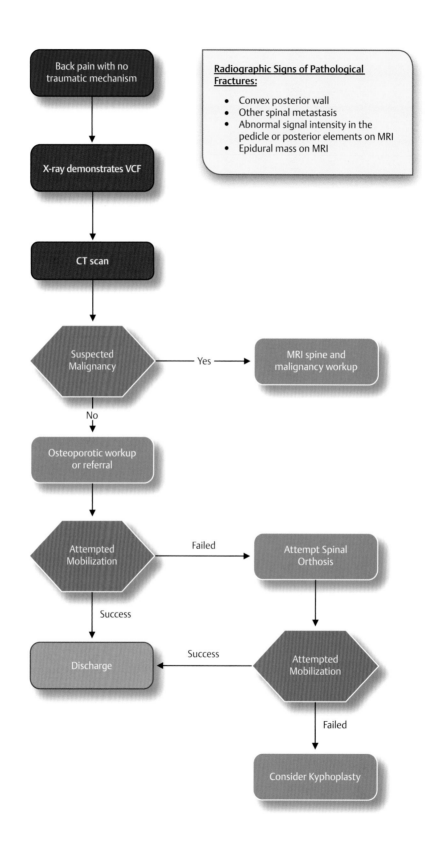

Suggested Readings

Jung et al 2003 Radiographics Volume 23 Number 1, Discrimination of Metastatic From Acute Osteoporotic Compression Spinal Fractures with MR Imaging

Safety and efficacy of vertebroplasty for acute painful osteoporotic fractures (VAPOUR): a multicentre, randomised, double-blind, placebo-controlled trial. 2016;388(10052):1408-1416.

Vertebroplasty and balloon kyphoplasty versus conservative treatment for osteoporotic vertebral compression fractures: A meta-analysis.

Jeremie Larouche, MD and R. Trigg McClellan, MD

Orthopaedic Trauma Institute
UCSF + SAN FRANCISCO GENERAL HOSPITAL

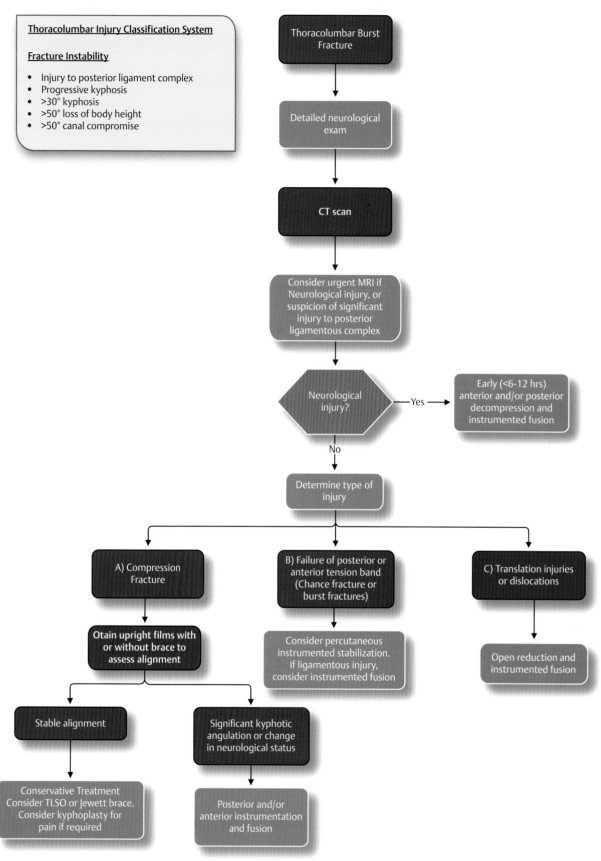

Thoracolumbar Injury Classification System

Fracture Instability

- Injury to posterior ligament complex
- Progressive kyphosis
- >30° kyphosis
- >50° loss of body height
- >50° canal compromise

Thoracolumbar Burst Fracture

Detailed neurological exam

CT scan

Consider urgent MRI if Neurological injury, or suspicion of significant injury to posterior ligamentous complex

Neurological injury? — Yes → Early (<6-12 hrs) anterior and/or posterior decompression and instrumented fusion

No

Determine type of injury

A) Compression Fracture

B) Failure of posterior or anterior tension band (Chance fracture or burst fractures)

C) Translation injuries or dislocations

Otain upright films with or without brace to assess alignment

Consider percutaneous instrumented stabilization. If ligamentous injury, consider instrumented fusion

Open reduction and instrumented fusion

Stable alignment

Significant kyphotic angulation or change in neurological status

Conservative Treatment Consider TLSO or Jewett brace. Consider kyphoplasty for pain if required

Posterior and/or anterior instrumentation and fusion

TLSO – Thoracolumbosacral Orthosis

Chapter 70: Bisphosphonate Femur Fractures

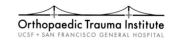

Eric Meinberg, MD

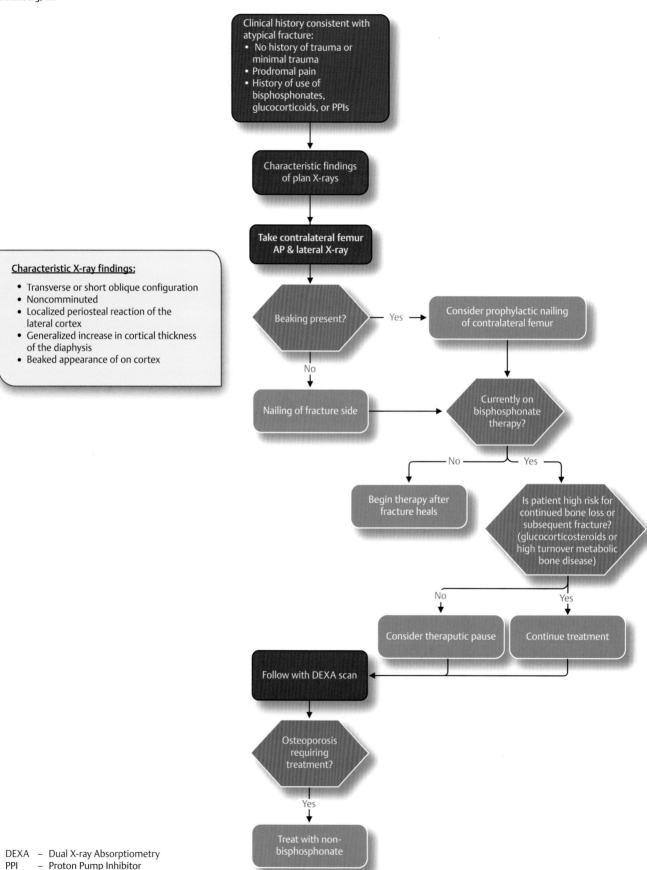

Characteristic X-ray findings:
- Transverse or short oblique configuration
- Noncomminuted
- Localized periosteal reaction of the lateral cortex
- Generalized increase in cortical thickness of the diaphysis
- Beaked appearance of on cortex

Clinical history consistent with atypical fracture:
- No history of trauma or minimal trauma
- Prodromal pain
- History of use of bisphosphonates, glucocorticoids, or PPIs

Characteristic findings of plan X-rays

Take contralateral femur AP & lateral X-ray

Beaking present? — Yes → Consider prophylactic nailing of contralateral femur

No ↓

Nailing of fracture side → Currently on bisphosphonate therapy?

No → Begin therapy after fracture heals

Yes → Is patient high risk for continued bone loss or subsequent fracture? (glucocorticosteroids or high turnover metabolic bone disease)

No → Consider theraputic pause

Yes → Continue treatment

Follow with DEXA scan

Osteoporosis requiring treatment?

Yes ↓

Treat with non-bisphosphonate

DEXA – Dual X-ray Absorptiometry
PPI – Proton Pump Inhibitor

Suggested Readings

Shane E, Burr D, Abrahamsen B, et al. Atypical subtrochanteric and diaphyseal femoral fractures: second report of a task force of the American Society for Bone and Mineral Research. J Bone Miner Res 2014;29(1):1–23

Chapter 71: Pathological (neoplastic) Fractures

Rosanna Wustrack, MD

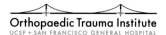
Suspected Pathologic Fracture

- Irregular fracture line
- Lytic/blastic lesion surrounding fracture site
- Known cancer diagnosis with metastatic potential

Aggressive Tumor Radiographic Characteristics

- Borders are ill-defined
- Cortical bone is destroyed
- Presence of Codman's triangle or periosteal reaction
- Surrounding soft tissue involvement

When to Biopsy?

- A lesion found on CT C/A/P with an unknown cancer diagnosis
- Solitary lesion or solitary skeletal metastasis
- To confirm suspected primary
- First bone metastases in a patient with a history of carcinoma

Prinicples of Fracture Fixation:

- Assume that fracture will not heal
- Maximize early mobilzation
- Consider embolization (esp. renal cell carcinoma)
- Consider adding PMMA to construct to replace pathologic bone
- Consider endoprosthetic replacement for peritrochanteric fractures for especially aggressive tumor types, ie renal cell.

CT C/A/P – CT of Chest, Abdomen and Pelvis
WBBS   – Whole Body Bone Scan
PMMA   – Polymethyl Methacrylate
MM   – Multiple Myeloma
SPEP   – Serum Protein Electrophoresis
UPEP   – Urine Protein Electrophoresis

Flowchart

Suspected pathological fracture on X-ray

↓

Radiographic lesion appears aggressive? — No →

↓ Yes

Thorough history and physical

↓

Send SPEP, UPEP and serum light chains to r/o MM

↓

Known cancer diagnosis? — No → **CT C/A/P and WBBS to look for primary malignancy and other skeletal metastases**

↓ Yes

Do lab findings and appearance match known neoplastic diagnosis?

(No branch →) **Biopsy most accessible bony lesion**

↓

CT C/A/P negative for primary lesion and WBBS negative for other skeletal metastases?

↓ Yes

Increased suspicion for primary bone sarcoma, refer to orthopedic oncologist.

↓ Yes (from "Do lab findings...")

Complete staging studies. If this is the FIRST bone metastasis, confirm with tissue diagnosis prior to definitive fixation. Can be done as image guided biopsy or as an open biopsy prior to fixation. If h/o renal cell carcinoma, refer to orthopedic oncologist.

↓

Complete fracture? — No → **Impending fracture? Lytic, proximal, >⅔ of diaphysis, painful?**

↓ Yes   ↓ Yes

Definitive fracture fixation ← Yes

↓

Consult with oncologist regarding adjuvant therapy — No

Suggested Readings

Rougraff BT, Kneisl JS, Simon MA. Skeletal metastases of unknown origin. A prospective study of a diagnostic strategy. J Bone Joint Surg Am. 1993 Sep;75(9):1276-81.

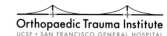

Paul Toogood, MD

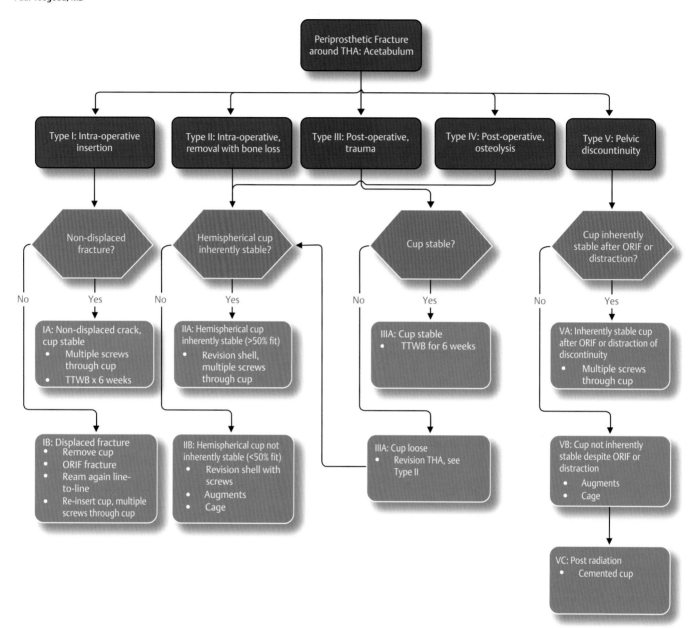

ORIF – Open Reduction Internal Fixation
TDWB – Touch Down Weight Bearing
THA – Total Hip Replacement

Suggested Readings

Della Valle CJ, Momberger NG, Paprosky WG. Periprosthetic fractures of the acetabulum associated with a total hip arthroplasty. Instr Course Lect 2003;52:281–290

Chapter 73: Periprosthetic Fracture around THA: Femur

Paul Toogood, MD

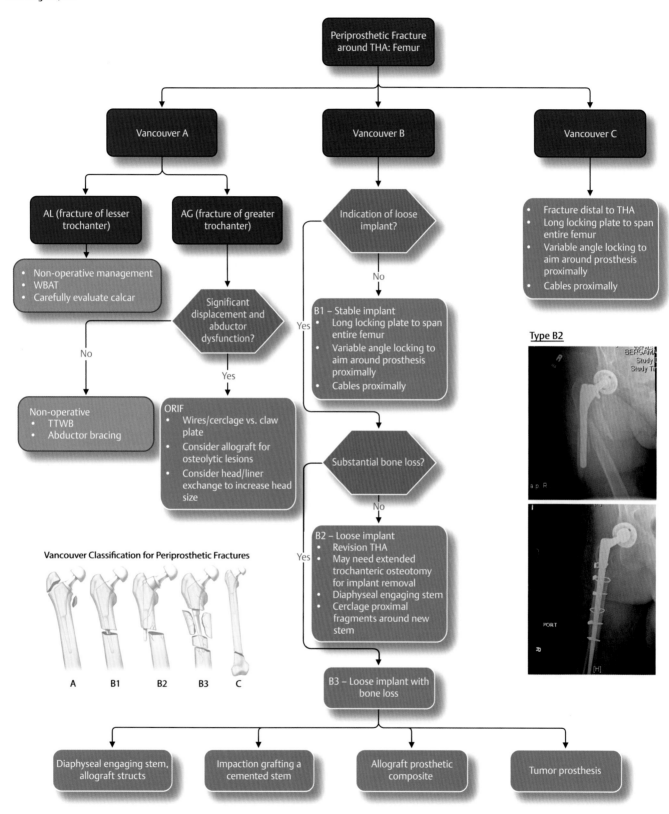

Periprosthetic Fracture around THA: Femur

Vancouver A

Vancouver B

Vancouver C
- Fracture distal to THA
- Long locking plate to span entire femur
- Variable angle locking to aim around prosthesis proximally
- Cables proximally

AL (fracture of lesser trochanter)
- Non-operative management
- WBAT
- Carefully evaluate calcar

AG (fracture of greater trochanter)

Significant displacement and abductor dysfunction?

No → Non-operative
- TTWB
- Abductor bracing

Yes → ORIF
- Wires/cerclage vs. claw plate
- Consider allograft for osteolytic lesions
- Consider head/liner exchange to increase head size

Indication of loose implant?

No → **B1 – Stable implant**
- Long locking plate to span entire femur
- Variable angle locking to aim around prosthesis proximally
- Cables proximally

Yes → Substantial bone loss?

No → **B2 – Loose implant**
- Revision THA
- May need extended trochanteric osteotomy for implant removal
- Diaphyseal engaging stem
- Cerclage proximal fragments around new stem

Yes → **B3 – Loose implant with bone loss**
- Diaphyseal engaging stem, allograft structs
- Impaction grafting a cemented stem
- Allograft prosthetic composite
- Tumor prosthesis

Type B2

Vancouver Classification for Periprosthetic Fractures

A   B1   B2   B3   C

THR – Total Hip Replacement
TTWB – Toe Touch Weight Bearing
WBAT – Weight Bearing As Tolerated

Suggested Readings

Brady OH, Garbuz DS, Masri BA, Duncan CP. Classification of the hip. Orthop Clin North Am 1999;30(2):215–220

Brady OH, Garbuz DS, Masri BA, Duncan CP. The reliability and validity of the Vancouver classification of femoral fractures after hip replacement. J Arthroplasty 2000;15(1):59–62

Chapter 74: Periprosthetic Fracture around TKA: Femur

Paul Toogood, MD

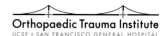
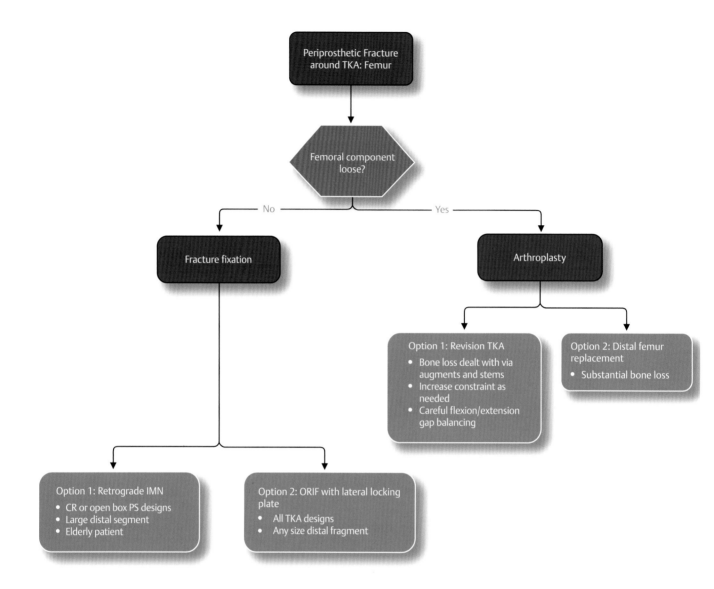

CR – Cruciate Retaining
PS – Posterior Stabilized
IMN – Intramedullary Nail
ORIF – Open Reduction Internal Fixation
TKA – Total Knee Replacement

Paul Toogood, MD

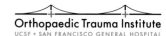

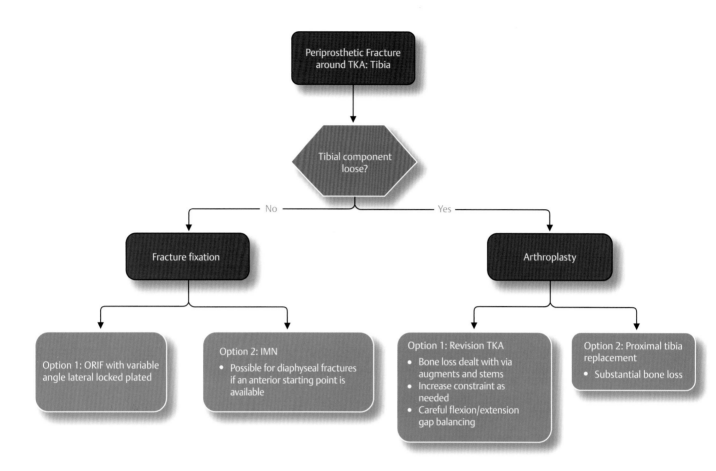

IMN – Intramedullary Nail
ORIF – Open Reduction Internal Fixation
TKA – Total Knee Replacement

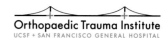

Meir T. Marmor, MD

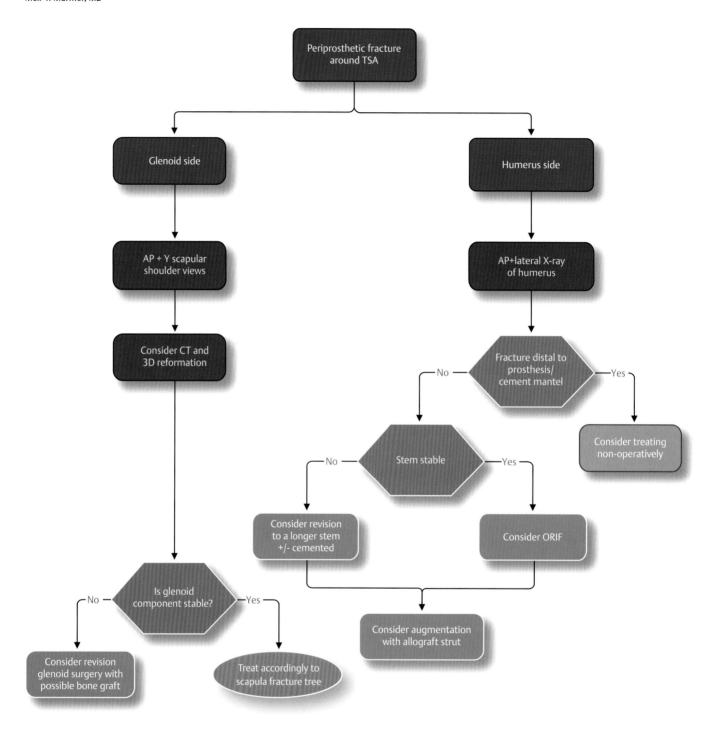

ORIF – Open Reduction and Internal Fixation

Suggested Readings

Kumar S, Sperling JW, Haidukewych GH, Cofield RH. Periprosthetic humeral fractures after shoulder arthroplasty. J Bone Joint Surg Am 2004;86-A(4):680–689

Hoffelner T, Moroder P, Auffarth A, Tauber M, Resch H. Outcomes after shoulder arthroplasty revision with glenoid reconstruction and bone grafting. Int Orthop 2014;38(4):775–782

Chapter 77: Fracture Delayed and Nonunion

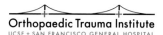

Theodore Miclau, MD

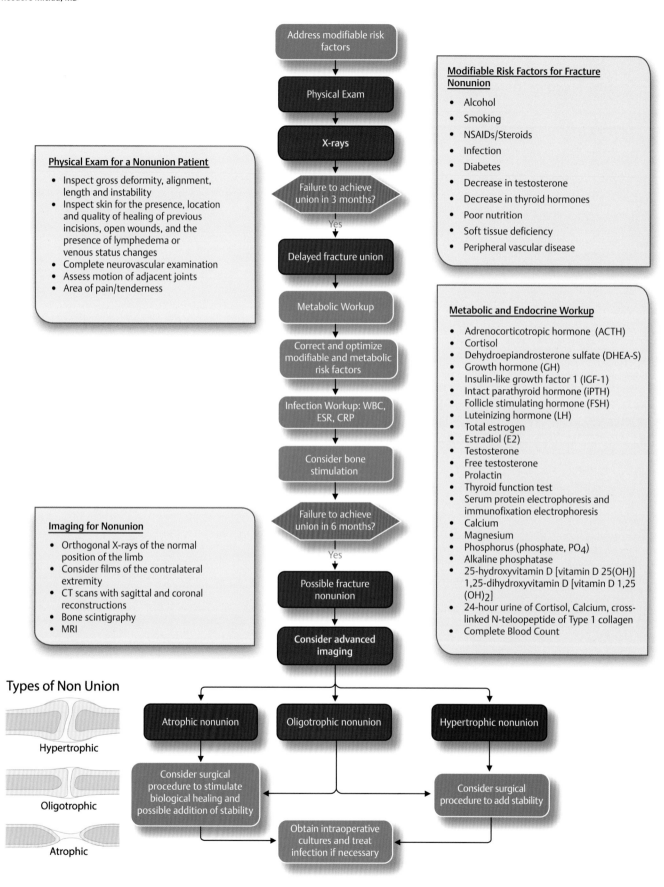

Address modifiable risk factors

Physical Exam

X-rays

Failure to achieve union in 3 months?
Yes

Delayed fracture union

Metabolic Workup

Correct and optimize modifiable and metabolic risk factors

Infection Workup: WBC, ESR, CRP

Consider bone stimulation

Failure to achieve union in 6 months?
Yes

Possible fracture nonunion

Consider advanced imaging

Atrophic nonunion

Oligotrophic nonunion

Hypertrophic nonunion

Consider surgical procedure to stimulate biological healing and possible addition of stability

Consider surgical procedure to add stability

Obtain intraoperative cultures and treat infection if necessary

Physical Exam for a Nonunion Patient

- Inspect gross deformity, alignment, length and instability
- Inspect skin for the presence, location and quality of healing of previous incisions, open wounds, and the presence of lymphedema or venous status changes
- Complete neurovascular examination
- Assess motion of adjacent joints
- Area of pain/tenderness

Imaging for Nonunion

- Orthogonal X-rays of the normal position of the limb
- Consider films of the contralateral extremity
- CT scans with sagittal and coronal reconstructions
- Bone scintigraphy
- MRI

Modifiable Risk Factors for Fracture Nonunion

- Alcohol
- Smoking
- NSAIDs/Steroids
- Infection
- Diabetes
- Decrease in testosterone
- Decrease in thyroid hormones
- Poor nutrition
- Soft tissue deficiency
- Peripheral vascular disease

Metabolic and Endocrine Workup

- Adrenocorticotropic hormone (ACTH)
- Cortisol
- Dehydroepiandrosterone sulfate (DHEA-S)
- Growth hormone (GH)
- Insulin-like growth factor 1 (IGF-1)
- Intact parathyroid hormone (iPTH)
- Follicle stimulating hormone (FSH)
- Luteinizing hormone (LH)
- Total estrogen
- Estradiol (E2)
- Testosterone
- Free testosterone
- Prolactin
- Thyroid function test
- Serum protein electrophoresis and immunofixation electrophoresis
- Calcium
- Magnesium
- Phosphorus (phosphate, PO_4)
- Alkaline phosphatase
- 25-hydroxyvitamin D [vitamin D 25(OH)] 1,25-dihydroxyvitamin D [vitamin D 1,25 $(OH)_2$]
- 24-hour urine of Cortisol, Calcium, cross-linked N-teloopeptide of Type 1 collagen
- Complete Blood Count

Types of Non Union

Hypertrophic

Oligotrophic

Atrophic

Suggested Readings

Brinker MR, O'Connor DP, Monla YT, Earthman TP. Metabolic and endocrine abnormalities in patients with nonunions. J Orthop Trauma 2007;21(8):557–570

Schenker ML, Wigner NA, Lopas L, Hankenson KD, Ahn J. Fracture repair and bone grafting. Orthopaedic Knowledge Update 2014;11:1–1

Chapter 78: Acute Surgical Infection

Harry Jergesen, MD

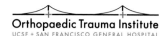

Orthopaedic Trauma Institute
UCSF + SAN FRANCISCO GENERAL HOSPITAL

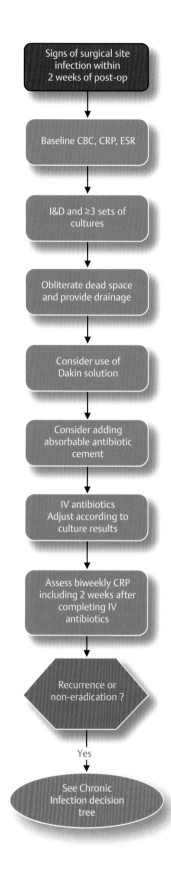

Signs of surgical site infection within 2 weeks of post-op

↓

Baseline CBC, CRP, ESR

↓

I&D and ≥3 sets of cultures

↓

Obliterate dead space and provide drainage

↓

Consider use of Dakin solution

↓

Consider adding absorbable antibiotic cement

↓

IV antibiotics Adjust according to culture results

↓

Assess biweekly CRP including 2 weeks after completing IV antibiotics

↓

Recurrence or non-eradication ?

Yes ↓

See Chronic Infection decision tree

Chapter 79: Post-Operative Chronic Infection

Harry Jergesen, MD

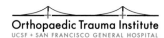

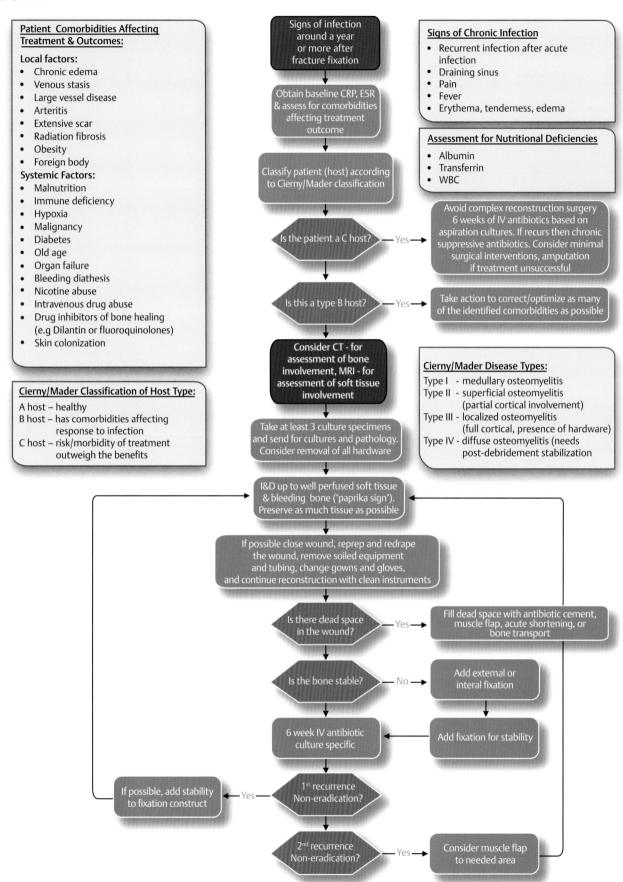

Patient Comorbidities Affecting Treatment & Outcomes:

Local factors:
- Chronic edema
- Venous stasis
- Large vessel disease
- Arteritis
- Extensive scar
- Radiation fibrosis
- Obesity
- Foreign body

Systemic Factors:
- Malnutrition
- Immune deficiency
- Hypoxia
- Malignancy
- Diabetes
- Old age
- Organ failure
- Bleeding diathesis
- Nicotine abuse
- Intravenous drug abuse
- Drug inhibitors of bone healing (e.g Dilantin or fluoroquinolones)
- Skin colonization

Cierny/Mader Classification of Host Type:

A host – healthy
B host – has comorbidities affecting response to infection
C host – risk/morbidity of treatment outweigh the benefits

Signs of infection around a year or more after fracture fixation

Obtain baseline CRP, ESR & assess for comorbidities affecting treatment outcome

Classify patient (host) according to Cierny/Mader classification

Is the patient a C host? —Yes→ Avoid complex reconstruction surgery 6 weeks of IV antibiotics based on aspiration cultures. If recurs then chronic suppressive antibiotics. Consider minimal surgical interventions, amputation if treatment unsuccessful

Is this a type B host? —Yes→ Take action to correct/optimize as many of the identified comorbidities as possible

Consider CT - for assessment of bone involvement, MRI - for assessment of soft tissue involvement

Take at least 3 culture specimens and send for cultures and pathology. Consider removal of all hardware

I&D up to well perfused soft tissue & bleeding bone ("paprika sign"). Preserve as much tissue as possible

If possible close wound, reprep and redrape the wound, remove soiled equipment and tubing, change gowns and gloves, and continue reconstruction with clean instruments

Is there dead space in the wound? —Yes→ Fill dead space with antibiotic cement, muscle flap, acute shortening, or bone transport

Is the bone stable? —No→ Add external or interal fixation → Add fixation for stability

6 week IV antibiotic culture specific

1st recurrence Non-eradication? —Yes→ If possible, add stability to fixation construct

2nd recurrence Non-eradication? —Yes→ Consider muscle flap to needed area

Signs of Chronic Infection
- Recurrent infection after acute infection
- Draining sinus
- Pain
- Fever
- Erythema, tenderness, edema

Assessment for Nutritional Deficiencies
- Albumin
- Transferrin
- WBC

Cierny/Mader Disease Types:

Type I   - medullary osteomyelitis
Type II - superficial osteomyelitis (partial cortical involvement)
Type III - localized osteomyelitis (full cortical, presence of hardware)
Type IV - diffuse osteomyelitis (needs post-debridement stabilization

Orthopaedic Trauma Institute
UCSF + SAN FRANCISCO GENERAL HOSPITAL

158

Suggested Readings

Cierny G III. Surgical treatment of osteomyelitis. Plast Reconstr Surg 2011;127(Suppl 1):190S–204S

Cierny G III, Mader JT, Penninck JJ. A clinical staging system for adult osteomyelitis. Clin Orthop Relat Res 2003; (414):7–24

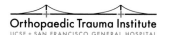

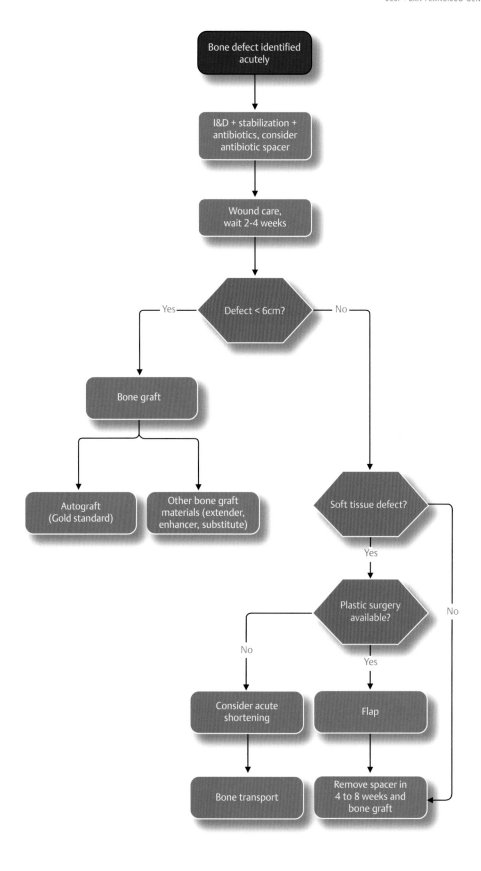

I&D – Irrigation and Debridement

Suggested Readings

Mauffrey C, Hake ME, Chadayammuri V, Masquelet AC. Reconstruction of Long Bone Infections Using the Induced Membrane Technique: Tips and Tricks. J Orthop Trauma 2016;30(6):e188–e193

Sen C, Kocaoglu M, Eralp L, Gulsen M, Cinar M. Bifocal compression-distraction in the acute treatment of grade III open tibia fractures with bone and soft-tissue loss: a report of 24 cases. J Orthop Trauma 2004;18(3):150–157

Sen MK, Miclau T. Autologous iliac crest bone graft: should it still be the gold standard for treating nonunions? Injury 2007;38(Suppl 1):S75–S80 Review

Appendix A: Imaging

Chapter	Extremity emergencies	Author	X-rays	Advance imaging
15	Traumatic Anterior Shoulder Instability	Lee	Shoulder AP, axillary and transscapular Y	CT & MR arthrogram
16	Acromioclavicular Separation	Marmor	Bilateral AP, axillary, and Zanca views of the shoulder	
17	Sternoclavicular Dislocation (SCD)	Kandemir	Serendipity (40° cephalad tilt)	CT angio or MRA of upper chest
18	Clavicle Fractures	Toogood	Shoulder AP, scapular Y, and lateral Clavicle AP and cephalic tilt	CT scan (for medial 1/3 fractures)
19	Scapulothoracic Dissociation (STD)	Kandemir	Chest	CTA/MRA
20	Scapula Fractures	Kandemir	Dedicated shoulder radiographs to better visualize the scapula (i.e. Grashey, scapular Y, axillary) Large cassette to include whole scapula	CT with 3D reconstruction for accurate measurements if significant displacement is identified on plain radiographs
21	Proximal Humerus Fractures	Kandemir	Grashey, scapular Y, and axillary view	CT scan with 3D reconstruction
22	Humeral Shaft Fractures	Toogood	AP & lateral views of humerus, elbow, and shoulder	
23	Distal Humerus Fractures	Toogood	AP & lateral views of elbow	Consider CT with thin cuts + 2D & 3D reconstruction
24	Elbow Dislocation/ Terrible Triad Injury	Kandemir	AP, lateral, and radial head view	CT scan with 3D reconstruction
25	Radial Head Fractures	Lee	AP & lateral views, radiocapitellar views	CT scan
26	Capitellum Fractures	Kandemir	AP, lateral, and radial head view	CT scan with 3D reconstruction
27	Olecranon Fractures	Lee	AP, lateral elbow	CT scan
28	Forearm Fractures	Lee	AP & lateral X-ray of forearm Contralateral forearm and wrist X-rays to measure: radial bow, ulnar variance	
29	Distal Radius Fractures	Lee	AP, lateral, oblique wrist X-ray	CT scan
30	Scaphoid Fractures	Schroeder	AP, lateral, oblique wrist and scaphoid view (ulnar deviation)	
31	Perilunate Dislocation	Lee	PA and lateral wrist view	CT scan
32	Extensor Tendon Lacerations	Schroeder	AP view of hand	
33	Flexor Tendon Injuries	Schroeder	AP view of hand	
34	Finger Replantation	Schroeder	AP, lateral, oblique views of hand and amputated digit	
35	Finger Fractures	Schroeder	AP, lateral, oblique views	
36	Metacarpal Fractures	Schroeder	AP, lateral, oblique hand views	
37	Metacarpophalangeal (MCP) Dislocations	Schroeder	AP, lateral, oblique hand views	
38	Phalanx Dislocations	Schroeder	AP & true lateral views of all finger joints	

Chapter	Extremity emergencies	Author	X-rays	Advance imaging
LOWER EXTREMITY TRAUMA				
39	Femoral Shaft Fractures	McClellan	AP & lateral views of the femur	CT scan to rule out femoral neck fracture
40	Distal Femur Fractures	Toogood	AP & lateral views of knee AP & lateral views of femur	CT scan
41	Traumatic Knee Dislocation	Kandemir	AP & lateral views	CT angio, MRI, or MRA if vascular injury suspected
42	Patella Fractures	Marmor	AP, lateral, and skyline views of the knee	
43	Tibia Plateau Fractures	Morshed	AP & lateral views of the knee	CT scan with thin cuts 2D and 3D reconstructions
44	Tibia Shaft Fractures	McClellan	AP & lateral views of the tibia AP & lateral X-rays of ipsilateral knee and ankle	CT scan to rule out articular extension
45	Tibia Plafond Fractures	McClellan	AP, lateral, & mortise views of the ankle 2 views of ipsilateral knee 3 views of ipsilateral foot	CT ankle with axial, coronal, and sagittal cuts
46	Ankle Fractures	Marmor	AP, lateral, and mortise views of the ankle, Gravity stress view to test deltoid competency	Consider CT scan for posterior malleolus fractures or for fractures extending to the tibial plafond
47	Talus Fractures	Shearer	AP & lateral view of foot AP, lateral & mortise of ankle	CT scan of foot with thin cuts and 2D reconstructions
48	Calcaneus Fractures	Coughlin	AP & lateral foot views Harris heel view	CT scan of calcaneus with thin axial cuts and 2D reconstruction per standard protocol (coronal sections are perpendicular to posterior facet (~30 degrees), transverse sections perpendicular to coronal sections, regular sagittal sections)
49	Lisfranc Fractures	Shearer	AP, oblique, lateral foot views Bilateral weight bearing views	CT scan of foot with thin cuts and 2D reconstructions
50	Navicular Fractures	Shearer	AP, oblique, lateral foot views	CT scan of foot with thin cuts and 2D reconstructions
51	Metatarsal Fractures	Shearer	AP, oblique, lateral foot views	
52	Toe Fractures	Shearer	AP, oblique, lateral foot views	
	PELVIS AND HIP TRAUMA			
53	Pelvic Ring Fractures	Matityahu	AP, Inlet & Outlet views of the pelvis	CT scan with thin cuts 2D and 3D reconstructions
54	Acetabulum Fractures	Matityahu	AP and Judet views of the pelvis	CT scan with thin cuts 2D and 3D reconstructions
55	Hip Dislocations	Matityahu	AP pelvis, cross table lateral of hip	CT scan with thin cuts 2D
56	Femoral Head Fractures	Matityahu	AP, lateral of hip, AP pelvis with Judet views	CT scan with thin cuts 2D MRI
57	Intertrochanteric Fractures	Shearer	Pelvis AP view Hip AP & lateral view Femur AP & lateral view	
58	Femoral Neck Fractures	Meinberg	AP view of pelvis and hip Lateral view of hip AP & lateral views of ipsilateral femur	
59	Femoral Subtrochanteric Fractures	Shearer	Pelvis AP view Hip AP & lateral view Femur AP & lateral view	

Chapter	Extremity emergencies	Author	X-rays	Advance imaging
SPINE TRAUMA				
60	Spinal Cord Injury (SCI)	Larouche/ McClellan		CT MRI
61	Adult C-Spine Clearance after Blunt Trauma	Larouche/ McClellan		Cervical CT scan with coronal and sagittal reconstruction MRI
62	Occipitocervical Dissociations	Larouche/ McClellan		CT and CTA MRI with STIR
63	Atlas (C1) Fractures and Transverse Ligament Injuries	Larouche/ McClellan		CT scan +/− CTA if vertebral artery injury suspected
64	C2 Odontoid (dens) Fractures	Larouche/ McClellan	Flexion-extension views after 12 weeks in cervical orthosis	CT scan
65	C2 Traumatic Spondylolisthesis	Larouche/ McClellan		CT scan +/− CT angio if vertebral artery is suspected Consider MRI to assess integrity of C2/3 disc if necessary
66	C3-C7 Facet Dislocations	Larouche/ McClellan		Immediate CT and CTA for assessment of vertebral arteries and neurological exam Urgent MRI to assess for disc herniation or canal compromise
67	C3-C7 Lateral Mass Fractures	Larouche/ McClellan		CT and CTA to assess for vertebral artery injury MRI to assess disc integrity ALL PLL
68	Geriatric Vertebral Compression Fracture (VCF)	Larouche/ McClellan	AP, lateral views of thoracic and lumbar spine	CT scan
69	Thoracolumbar Fractures	Larouche/ McClellan	AP, lateral views of thoracic and lumbar spine	CT scan

Below is a summary of all the non-operative and rehabilitation recommendations mentioned throughout this book. These recommendations should not be applied uniformly, as injuries in a specific patient may be variable. The reader is should consult the treating orthopaedic surgeon or the surgical note for more specific recommendations for a given patient.

Appendix B: Rehabilitation

Chapter	Extremity emergencies	Author	Possible non-operative rehabilitation	Possible post-operative rehabilitation
15	Traumatic Anterior Shoulder Instability	Lee	Sling for 1 week Begin active ROM at 1 week	Per surgical note
16	Acromioclavicular Separation	Marmor	Same as operative	Sling for comfort Weight bearing up to 5lb for 6 weeks Early active range of motion, try to regain full range of motion in 6 weeks Return to normal activity in 12 weeks
17	Sternoclavicular Dislocation (SCD)	Kandemir	Sling for comfort NWB 6 weeks Pendulum exercises 1-2 weeks Active ROM as tolerated afterwards Start gradual WB at 6 weeks	Same as non-operative
18	Clavicle Fractures	Toogood	Sling/NWB for 6 weeks Elbow, wrist, finger ROM Pendulum exercises for 4 weeks (any ROM allowed below 90 of shoulder flexion/abduction) then AROM for 4 to 6 weeks At 6 weeks WBAT and full ROM	Immediate full passive or active ROM Sling in public places At 6 weeks WBAT
20	Scapula Fractures	Kandemir	First 6 weeks: Sling for comfort, full active or passive ROM After 6 weeks: gradual increase of weight bearing and activities	Immediate active and passive ROM, NWB After 6 weeks: Begin strengthening and resistance with gradual increase in weights After 12 weeks: Begin full strength and endurance program
21	Proximal Humerus Fractures	Kandemir	Shoulder brace with pillow for 6 weeks Start pendulum exercises at 10-14 days Start active & active assisted range of motion at 2 weeks Start passive range of motion at 6 weeks Start resisted exercises at 12 weeks	Shoulder brace with pillow for 6 weeks Start pendulum exercises postop day #1 Start active and active assisted range of motion postop day #1 Start passive range of motion at 6 weeks Start resisted exercises at 12 weeks
22	Humeral Shaft Fractures	Toogood	Coaptation splint Sarmiento brace at 1 week with films in brace1 Films every 1 to 2 weeks to check alignment until fracture "sticky" (less mobile on exam) Discontinue brace when fracture stable on exam and pain controlled WBAT when films show 3 of 4 cortices united	Immediate full ROM Okay to perform ADLs (<5lbs) WBAT when: Pain controlled; 3 of 4 cortices healed; if fracture bridged 12 weeks if compression plating
23	Distal Humerus Fractures	Toogood	Same as operative	Splint ~3 days to allow incision to heal Full ROM, NWB for 12 weeks once splint is removed Full ROM, WBAT after 12 weeks (except TEA, which has lifetime 5lbs weight limit)

Chapter	Extremity emergencies	Author	Possible non-operative rehabilitation	Possible post-operative rehabilitation
24	Elbow Dislocation/ Terrible Triad Injury	Kandemir	Elbow stable at full range of motion: Sling for comfort for 1-2 weeks Indomethacin for heterotopic ossification prophylaxis Non-weight bearing for 6 months Start range of motion exercises day #1 Elbow stable only at 30 degrees to full flexion: Hinged elbow brace 30°-full flexion at 1-2 weeks Gradual increase of extension at 3-4 weeks Non-weight bearing for 3 months Strengthening at 3 months Indomethacin for Heterotopic ossification prophylaxis	Per surgical note
25	Radial Head Fractures	Lee	Similar to operative	Sling for comfort NWB 6 weeks Active and passive ROM exercises
26	Capitellum Fractures	Kandemir	Non-weight bearing Gradual increase of range of motion Hinged elbow brace start range of motion exercises day #1	Non-weight bearing 6 weeks Full range of motion Start range of motion exercises day #1
27	Olecranon Fractures	Lee	Immobilize for 2 weeks ROM 0-90° for 4 weeks Free ROM 4-6 weeks	Splint for 2 weeks Remove posterior long arm splint and stitches at 2 weeks Begin AROM of elbow and forearm pronosupination, NWB 0-6 weeks At 6 weeks, WBAT and begin PROM in addition to AROM
28	Forearm Fractures	Lee	Forearm Clamshell brace for 6 weeks	NWB for 6 weeks Full ROM for 6 weeks
29	Distal Radius Fractures	Lee	Week 1: X-rays in sugar tong Overwrap sugar tong with fiberglass for snug fit Week 2: X-rays in splint Assess reduction Week 3: X-rays in splint Assess reduction If acceptable, transition to SAC for 3 weeks Week 6: X-rays out of cast WBAT Removable wrist splint and wean out over 2 weeks	Remove postop splint and stitches at 1 week Transition to removable wrist splint and being AROM of wrist and forearm, NWB 0-6 weeks At 6 weeks, WBAT and transition out of brace
30	Scaphoid Fractures	Schroeder	Distal pole - Thumb Spica cast, 4-6 weeks Waist - Thumb Spica cast, 8-12 weeks	Non weight bearing for 6-8 weeks, per surgeon.
31	Perilunate Dislocation	Lee		Per surgeon's guidelines
32	Extensor Tendon Laceration	Schroeder	If <60% of tendon width, ROM allowed	Depends on zone of injury, follow surgeon's guidelines
33	Flexor Tendon Injuries	Schroeder		Dorsal block splint with wrist flexed 10-20° MPs flexed 70° and IPs resting ROM per surgeon's guidelines
34	Finger Replantation	Schroeder		Per surgeon's guidelines
35	Finger Fractures	Schroeder	For stable fractures, buddy tape and early ROM	Per surgeon's guidelines
36	Metacarpal Fractures	Schroeder	Early ROM exercises	Early motion for stable internal fixation Casting for 4 weeks for CRPP, move IPs immediately.

Chapter	Extremity emergencies	Author	Possible non-operative rehabilitation	Possible post-operative rehabilitation
37	Metacarpophalangeal (MCP) Dislocations	Schroeder	Dorsal blocking splint with wrist extended 20° MPs fully flexed and IPs free Begin IP motion immediately	Per surgeon's guidelines
38	Phalanx Dislocations	Schroeder	DIP dislocation - gentle ROM once reduced PIP dorsal dislocation - buddy tape to adjacent finger, begin early ROM PIP volar dislocation - PIP splint in full extension for 6 weeks	Per surgeon's guidelines
LOWER EXTREMITY TRAUMA				
39	Femoral Shaft Fractures	McClellan		WBAT as tolerated for stable fracture patterns (Winquist 0-1) TDWB for unstable patterns (Winquist 2-4) Progress to WBAT at 6 weeks Knee ROM and quad strengthening at 2 weeks
40	Distal Femur Fractures	Toogood	Same as operative	12 weeks NWB with FROM exercises WBAT after 12 weeks
41	Traumatic Knee Dislocation	Kandemir	Hinged knee brace for 6-12 weeks Hinged knee brace locked in extension for 1 week then ROM exercises in brace	Expectant management: Discontinue external fixator at 4-6 weeks Start range of motion in hinged knee brace Reevaluate at 3 months Early repair - per surgical note
42	Patella Fractures	Marmor	FWB only in extension brace/cast Isometric quad exercise ASAP Resistance exercises at 6 weeks (avoid active extension until 6 weeks Progressive ROM from weeks 2-6 at specified intervals, e.g. 15 degree increments per week Consider immobilization	Hinged knee brace for 8 weeks Full weight bearing only with brace locked in extension for 8 weeks For stable fixation – passive ROM 0-30 in first 4 weeks and advance by 15 degrees every week afterwards For tenuous fixation – extension brace/cast for 6 weeks
43	Tibia Plateau Fractures	Morshed	Initial non-operative treatment: Non-weight bearing for 6 weeks Hinged knee brace Early range of motion after 6 weeks: Hinged knee brace Mobilization and graduated weight bearing and walking	NWB for 6 weeks Partial progressive weight bearing for 6 weeks Full active and passive ROM Hinged knee brace if there is accompanying cruciate or collateral ligament injury
44	Tibia Shaft Fractures	McClellan	Long leg cast for 4 weeks Convert to functional cast brace (Sarmiento) until fracture union Weight bearing as tolerated after 4 weeks & X-ray follow-up every 2 weeks	2 weeks in a posterior splint with the foot plantigrade (ankle at 90) ROM knee and ankle at 2 weeks WBAT at 2 weeks for stable fracture patterns NWB 6 weeks for unstable fracture patterns
45	Tibia Plafond (Pilon) Fractures	McClellan		Splint for 2-3 weeks Nonweight bearing for 12 weeks Passive and active range of motion at 2-3 weeks
46	Ankle Fractures	Marmor	WBAT for in CAM boot for 6 weeks For stable injuries 6-12 weeks NWB in short leg cast for unstable injuries	Splint 2 weeks WBAT in CAM boot and ROM exercises 4 weeks Syndesmosis injury - NWB 12 weeks, full ROM exercises Diabetic / severe osteoporosis : NWB 12 weeks Cast 6 weeks Full active and passive ROM exercises 6-12 weeks

Chapter	Extremity emergencies	Author	Possible non-operative rehabilitation	Possible post-operative rehabilitation
47	Talus Fractures	Shearer	Short leg cast for 6 weeks then progressive weight bearing 25% every week	Well padded splint for 2 weeks Begin ankle and foot ROM 2 weeks after surgery For neck & body fractures - 12 weeks NWB For process fractures - 6 weeks NWB Progressive weight bearing afterwards (advance by 25% every week)
48	Calcaneus Fractures	Coughlin	Same as operative	NWB 6-12 weeks Early ROM (after 2 weeks)
49	Lisfranc Fractures	Shearer	Stable ligamentous injuries: CAM boot WBAT for 6 weeks Non-displaced bony Lisfranc injuries: Cast NWB for 6 weeks	Splint for 2 weeks, then CAM boot, begin ankle/subtalar motion Progressive weight bearing at 8 weeks (25% per week) K-wire removal at 6 to 8 weeks Screw removal at 3 to 6 months Return to sports 9 to 12 months
50	Navicular Fractures	Shearer	Cast for 6 weeks NWB	ORIF: Splint for 2 weeks then CAM boot, ankle and subtalar ROM NWB for 8 weeks then progressive weight bearing (25%/week) Ex-fix: removal at 6 weeks, NWB 3 months Bridge plate: removal at 3-4 months, NWB 3 months
51	Metatarsal Fractures	Shearer	1st Metatarsal - NWB cast for 6 weeks 2-4th Metatarsals - Stiff sole postop shoe or boot for 6 weeks WBAT 5th metatarsal: Zone 1 - Stiff sole shoe or boot for 6 weeks WBAT Zone 2/3 - NWB cast for 6 weeks	Per surgical note 5th MT Zone 2/3 can begin early weight bearing after IM stabilization
52	Toe Fractures	Shearer	Heel weight bearing stiff sole shoe	Heel weight bearing stiff sole shoe

PELVIS AND HIP TRAUMA

Chapter	Extremity emergencies	Author	Possible non-operative rehabilitation	Possible post-operative rehabilitation
53	Pelvic Ring Fractures	Matityahu	WBAT for stable injuries	TDWB 6-12 weeks Early ROM
54	Acetabulum Fractures	Matityahu	WBAT for stable injuries	TDWB 6-12 weeks Early ROM
55	Hip Dislocations	Matityahu	WBAT for stable injuries	TDWB 6-12 weeks Early ROM
56	Femoral Head Fractures	Matityahu	TDWB for 6 weeks with restricted abduction for Pipkin I fractures	For Pipkin II-IV injuries: TDWB 3 months Hip abductor strengthening exercises After 3 months, WBAT and gait training
57	Intertrochanteric Fractures	Shearer		Geriatric: WBAT Young: Depends on fracture pattern/fixation
58	Femoral Neck Fractures	Meinberg	For stable (valgus impacted) injuries - WBAT Otherwise TDWB	Arthroplasty - WBAT ORIF - TDWB, early ROM
59	Femoral Subtrochanteric Fractures	Shearer		Geriatric: WBAT Young: Depends on fracture pattern/fixation

Appendix C: Orthoses

Chapter	Extremity emergencies	Author	Recommended orthoses	Comments
UPPER EXTREMITY TRAUMA				
15	Traumatic Anterior Shoulder Instability	Lee	Shoulder abduction brace or Airplane splint	
16	Acromioclavicular Separation	Marmor	Sling	
17	Sternoclavicular Dislocation (SCD)	Kandemir	Shoulder Immobilizer	
18	Clavicle Fractures	Toogood	Sling	
19	Scapulothoracic Dissociation (STD)	Kandemir	Shoulder Immobilizer	
20	Scapula Fractures	Kandemir	Shoulder Immobilizer or sling	
21	Proximal Humerus Fractures	Kandemir	Shoulder Immobilizer	
22	Humerus Shaft Fractures	Toogood	Sarmiento brace	Sling may be added
23	Distal Humerus Fractures	Toogood	None	
24	Elbow Dislocation/ Terrible Triad Injury	Kandemir	Elbow ROM (hinged) brace	If stable in full range of motion - no brace is needed
25	Radial Head Fractures	Lee	Elbow ROM brace	Sling may be added
26	Capitellum Fractures	Kandemir	None	
27	Olecranon Fractures	Lee	Elbow ROM brace	Sling may be added. Post-cast stabilization
28	Forearm Fractures	Lee	Forearm fracture brace	Sling may be added
29	Distal Radius Fractures	Lee	Forearm-wrist fracture brace	Wrist brace for healing fractures coming out of cast
30	Scaphoid Fractures	Schroeder	Thump spica orthosis	
31	Perilunate Dislocation	Lee		
32	Extensor Tendon Lacerations	Schroeder	Volar wrist and hand splint	
33	Flexor Tendon Injuries	Schroeder	Dorsal blocking splint	
34	Finger Replantation	Schroeder	Custom splint, depending on injury	
35	Finger Fractures	Schroeder	Finger splints	
36	Metacarpal Fractures	Schroeder	Short arm or boxers cast	
37	Metacarpophalangeal (MCP) Dislocations	Schroeder	Dorsal blocking splint	
38	Phalanx Dislocations	Schroeder	Finger splints	
LOWER EXTREMITY TRAUMA				
39	Femoral Shaft Fractures	McClellan	None	
40	Distal Femur Fractures	Toogood	None	
41	Traumatic Knee Dislocation	Kandemir	Knee Immobilizer - initial treatment in emergency department Knee ROM (hinged) brace - after surgery	
42	Patella Fractures	Marmor	Knee Immobilizer	Followed by range of motion knee brace when beginning to mobilize
43	Tibia Plateau Fractures	Morshed	None	
44	Tibia Shaft Fractures	McClellan	Tibial fracture brace bivalve	With or without the ankle joint and foot extension

Chapter	Extremity emergencies	Author	Recommended orthoses	Comments
45	Tibia Plafond (Pilon) Fractures	McClellan	CAM Walker	After surgical fixation
46	Ankle Fractures	Marmor	CAM Walker	Well-padded splint for the first 2 weeks after surgery
47	Talus Fractures	Shearer	CAM Walker	For use when ready to begin ROM exercises, typically 2-6 weeks post-injury
48	Calcaneus Fractures	Coughlin	CAM Walker Ankle Foot Orthosis (AFO) for symptomatic malunions	Post-surgical possibly use rigid insert in the shoe
49	Lisfranc Fractures	Shearer	CAM Walker	For use when ready to begin ROM exercises, typically 2-6 weeks post-injury
50	Navicular Fractures	Shearer	CAM Walker	For use when ready to begin ROM exercises, typically 2-6 weeks post-injury
51	Metatarsal Fractures	Shearer	CAM Walker or post-op shoe	WBAT for 2-4th, 5th Zone 1
52	Toe Fractures	Shearer	Post-op shoe	Heel weight bearing if unstable

SPINE TRAUMA

Chapter	Extremity emergencies	Author	Recommended orthoses	Comments
60	Spinal Cord Injury (SCI)	Larouche, McClellan		
61	Adult C-Spine Clearance after Blunt Trauma	Larouche, McClellan		
62	Occipitocervical Dislocations	Larouche, McClellan		
63	Atlas (C1) Fractures and Transverse Ligament Injuries	Larouche, McClellan	HALO	
64	C2 Odontoid (dens) Fractures	Larouche, McClellan	HALO or cervical collar	Usually after surgical fixation
65	C2 Traumatic Spondylolisthesis	Larouche, McClellan	HALO or cervical collar	
66	C3-C7 Facet Dislocations	Larouche, McClellan	Cervical collar or CTO	Depending on level
67	C3-C7 Lateral Mass Fractures	Larouche, McClellan	Cervical collar or CTO	
68	Geriatric Vertebral Compression Fracture (VCF)	Larouche, McClellan	Jewett or TLSO	Depending on compartment
69	Thoracolumbar Injuries	Larouche, McClellan	Bivalve TLSO	

Appendix D: Estimated Time to Return to Work

The following chart should not be used to predict the time to return to work for a given patient. The chart is not validated for this purpose. Rather, the chart should be used only as the basis for a conversation with the patient on the amount of time before he or she can return to work. The chart can help the patient understand the factors that may influence the return to work time and together with his surgeon can devise a plan for returning to work.

The chart applies to all orthopaedic injuries at every given time after surgery.

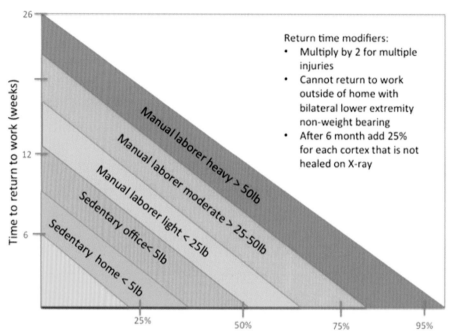

ROM – Range Of Motion

WB – Weight Bearing

% Functional recovery= (%Pain recovery + %ROM gain + %ability to bear weight + %muscle strength recovery) / 4

Examples for use of the chart:

- *Engineer with an ankle fracture*, *6 weeks after surgery, has 3/10 (pain (70% recovery), has regained 80% of his ROM compared to contralateral side, is able to place 100% of his weight on the ankle and has regained 50% of muscle strength = Sedentary office, 75% healing => <u>can return to work.</u>*

- *Motorcycle repairman that lifts more than 50lb at work with a tibia shaft fracture*, *10 weeks after surgery, has 7/10 pain (30% recovery), has regained 80% of his ROM compared to contralateral side, is able to place 100% of his weight on the leg and has regained 50% of muscle strength = Manual laborer heavy, 65% functional recovery => <u>estimated time to return to work is 6-12 weeks.</u>*

- *Manual worker at a high-tech company with a distal radius fracture*, *9 weeks after surgery, pain is 5/10 (50% recovery), has regained only 10% of her ROM compared to contralateral side, is able to lift only 5% the weight she is able to lift on the uninjured side and has regained 20% of muscle strength = Manual laborer light, 21.5% functional recovery => <u>estimated time to return to work is 6-10 weeks.</u>*